"Thank you, Steve. I loved it! You are a

"Drinking only raw vegetables and fruits seemed to supercharge my taste buds, and I appreciate my food now so much more. I'm also much more picky about what I'm putting into my mouth!"

"Having done three juice cleanses since January, I'm almost at my ideal weight. I haven't been able to get back to that point in about six years."

"I just want to say thank you for being such a beautiful human being, bringing health back to all of us."

"I had never tried fasting of any kind, but after reading about Bill Clinton's amazing turnaround, he looks GREAT. Your detox class seemed like the right way to jump-start into a new way to eat, stay healthy, and lose weight. And I was right."

"Not only did I learn the correct and beneficial way to detox, I also learned some wonderful things that I can do daily that will help me attain better health!"

"From those seven days, I've learned how much I enjoy drinking veggies, rather than eating them!"

"I've tried many things and this is the only thing I keep coming back to. It always makes me feel better when I feel sick and downtrodden. Steve Meyerowitz is by far the BEST teacher in this field."

Sproutman's 7-Day

JUST JUICE DIET

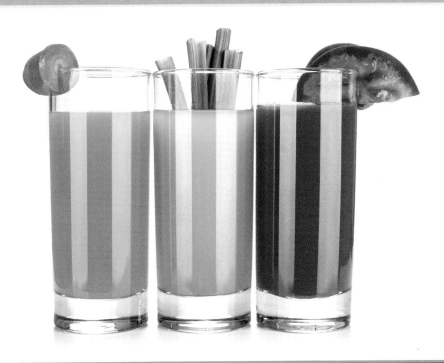

Steve Meyerowitz

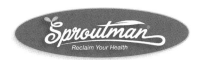

Healthy Living Publications
Summertown, Tennessee

Library of Congress Cataloging-in-Publication Data

Meyerowitz, Steve.
  Sproutman's 7-day just juice diet : detox, lose weight, feel great / Steve Meyerowitz.
    pages cm
  Includes index.
  ISBN 978-1-57067-306-1 (pbk.) — ISBN 978-1-57067-878-3 (e-book)
  1. Fruit juices--Therapeutic use.   2. Vegetable juices—Therapeutic
use. 3. Beverages—Therapeutic use. 4. Herbs—Therapeutic use.   5. Raw
foods—Therapeutic use.   6. Detoxification (Health) 7. Weight loss. I. Title.
  RM255.M489 2014
  641.3'4—dc23

                                   2014026801

Disclaimer: The information in this book is not intended as medical advice, treatment, or therapy for any condition, and the information and recipes contained herein are not substitutes for treatment by a qualified health care professional. If you have any questions about your health, please consult a physician.

Cover and interior design: John Wincek
Stock photography: 123 RF

Printed in the United States of America

Healthy Living Publications,
An imprint of Book Publishing Company
P.O. Box 99
Summertown, TN 38483
888-260-8458
bookpubco.com

ISBN 13: 978-1-57067-306-1

20 19 18 17 16 15 14   1 2 3 4 5 6 7 8 9

Book Publishing Company is a member of Green Press Initiative. We chose to print this title on FSC certified paper with 10% postconsumer recycled content, processed without chlorine, which saves the following natural resources:

   10 trees
   293 pounds of solid waste
   4,377 gallons of water
   807 pounds of greenhouse gases
   4 million BTU of energy

For more information on Green Press Initiative, visit greenpressinitiative.org.

Environmental impact estimates were made using the Environmental Defense Fund Paper Calculator. For more information, visit papercalculator.org.

Printed on recycled paper

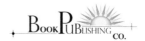

Contents

Introduction   vii

CHAPTER **1**

Juicing to Lose Weight, Detox, and Feel Great   1

CHAPTER **2**

Getting Started with the 7-Day Just Juice Diet   15

CHAPTER **3**

Selecting the Right Juicer and Juicing Efficiently   29

CHAPTER **4**

Planning Your Daily Routine   39

CHAPTER **5**

Optimizing Your Detoxification   53

CHAPTER **6**

Transitioning Back to Solid Food   71

CHAPTER **7**

Fighting for Your Health   87

CHAPTER **8**

Recipes   93

Resources   125

Index   129

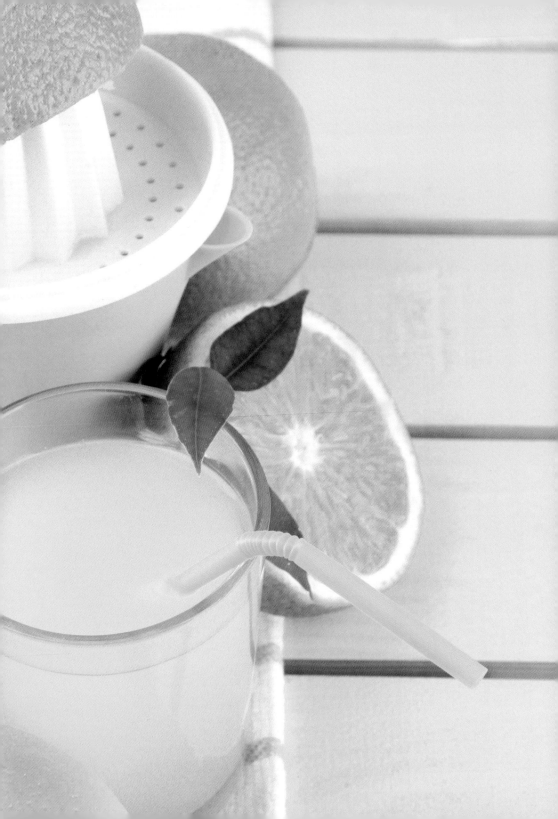

Introduction

I'm getting fired up for another week of just juice. I do this a few times every year. (Yes, it gets easier the more you do it.) Why? I love the way it makes me feel! I invest a week, and I collect dividends for months. The dividends I'm talking about are the kind that restore your natural energy and lighten your load. This happens when your body is cleaner and functions more efficiently. It's not a pricey pill; it's not a million-dollar secret. It's a 7-day protocol that requires commitment and discipline. I give you the recipes (they're delicious) and the daily program (it's flexible), and you make the commitment.

When I started my quest for healing in the 1970s, I'd been struggling with a lifetime of food sensitivities, constipation, asthma, and severe allergies to common things, such as animals, dust, and grass. Even breathing was hard! I discovered juice fasting and did a lot of it, even fasting for as long as one hundred days. I made so many mistakes! But I was determined to get it right and learned a great deal as I refined my process.

The program in this book is modeled after my work with thousands of students. Over the years, I've taught many classes, including international webinars. I lead groups through the 7-Day Just Juice Diet four to six times per year. And now I can help you—not just to avoid the pitfalls but also to get the greatest benefit from juice fasting in the shortest amount of time.

Even though this diet is about cleansing the body, the key to success is getting in the right frame of mind. Once you make the mental commitment, it's easier to deal with the challenges of the physical process. That's why I'll ask you to think about your goals first, and then I'll help you get organized.

This cleanse is not going to cure everything. One week of just juice can't reverse health issues that have developed over the course of a lifetime. However, cleansing naturally reduces inflammation, neutralizes allergies, purifies the bloodstream, purges the intestinal tract, balances the body's biochemistry, and yes, successfully eliminates unnecessary pounds. And here's the payoff: when you feel better in your body, you approach all your challenges with fresh energy and renewed enthusiasm.

If you take a break from the energy-consuming process of digestion, and from the contaminants in our modern food supply, your body will revert to its natural equilibrium. You'll recapture some of your old self, feeling more energetic and productive, and probably having a better memory and renewed ability to focus. And you can do this simply by peeling back the layers to become the best version of yourself. If it's done right, the Just Juice Diet is the fastest path to rejuvenation. Think of your body as a car and the diet as a tune-up. After seven days, you'll still be driving the same car, but you'll be getting better mileage and a smoother ride.

When you feel better in your body, you approach all your challenges with fresh energy and renewed enthusiasm.

In these pages you'll find answers to the most common questions I've gotten from folks who've already gone through the Just Juice Diet with me. So, think of this book as a road map and a support system that will keep you on track, just as if I were there with you.

Steve Meyerowitz

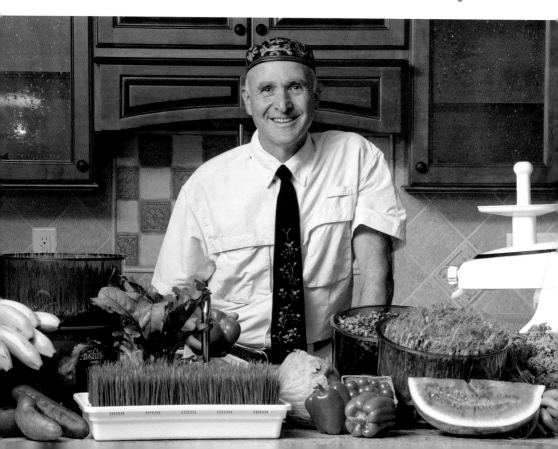

1

Juicing to Lose Weight, Detox, and Feel Great

Fasting has a long tradition. It's a part of every major religion: Buddha, Jesus, Moses, and Muhammad all fasted. Religious fasting means abstaining from all food and taking only water. Modern society doesn't have much of an appetite for this type of fasting, despite its ancient past. Because we live in such a food-oriented society, many folks just can't muster the willpower to do without their favorite foods for even a few days. Rest assured that the 7-Day Just Juice Diet is thoroughly nourishing and completely satisfying. Drinking vegetable juice is like drinking a salad! The menu for this juice fast includes nearly everything that grows on the ground or hangs from a tree. Far from abstinence, this kind of fasting is more like feasting!

Maybe you've noticed how exhausted you feel after a big meal. Your body is so busy laboring over everything you've put in it, it never gets a chance to catch up on housecleaning. That's why spending a week on just juice is exactly what you need. The phytochemicals (plant chemicals) in juiced fruits and vegetables act as natural detergents, scrubbing away at your insides. You'll feel lighter (in fact, you will be) and you'll feel younger because of the energy you saved by not engaging in the ordeal of digestion. Also, once you turn off your digestive furnace, the fog will lift and your mind will be quicker and clearer.

What are you going to do with this extra energy? Give it to your gallbladder. Flush your bile ducts. Stop those liver spots before they turn into stones. Unclog every artery and vessel. Conserve your energy for all this inner cleaning and you'll feel like a million bucks!

WHAT IS THE SPROUTMAN 7-DAY JUST JUICE DIET?

This is a one-week cleanse that's based on a flexible menu of raw vegetable juices, fruit juices (especially citrus), water, clear vegetable broths, herbal teas, and optional exotic drinks. I also recommend taking powerful probiotics to rebuild your intestinal terrain. This diet also includes techniques for detoxifying your liver and colon. In addition to cleaning you out, juices nourish you more thoroughly than solid foods. Your body digests, absorbs, and assimilates juice far more efficiently than it does solid food.

In following my program, you'll be exercising daily and will have the option to do some additional therapies, such as colonics, enemas, saunas or steam baths, and skin cleansing—all of which will enhance the healing process. These therapies are optional; you can pick and choose whatever works for you. However, I strongly encourage you to try as many of these therapies as you can to promote the cleansing and rejuvenation of your internal organs and get the best results.

The Just Juice Diet could be described as a cleanse or a "fast," a term that many people associate with hunger. I want to assure you that you're *not* going to be hungry. This is everyone's biggest fear when they consider going on a fast. Fasting is not starving. In fact, I promise that you'll be absorbing more nutrients and be better nourished this week by drinking a variety of juices than you would be by eating your usual diet. Oh, sure, maybe you'll miss eating food the first day or two, but that's to be expected and is completely manageable. After that . . . you're on easy street.

Normally, 80 percent of your available energy is spent on digesting and eliminating food. You'll be absolutely amazed at how good you feel once you're liberated from this daily process. How do I know? Countless students have told me! They've reported that they feel a brightness of spirit and a lightness in their step.

What Makes Up the 7-Day Just Juice Diet?

You can think of this diet as a cleanse or a juice fast. Whatever you call it, you'll find it brings renewed vitality. The program includes the following:

- a generous 7-day diet of raw vegetable and fruit juices
- colon-cleansing drinks, liver-cleansing drinks, herbal teas, and many optional drinks
- exercises and treatments to cleanse the liver, intestinal tract, lungs, bladder, kidneys, and skin

WHAT WILL A 7-DAY JUICE DIET DO FOR YOU?

F asting is a process of purification. Depending on how closely you follow this program, you can expect to achieve some level of blood purification, colon cleansing, and liver detoxification. All of this will have a positive and immeasurable impact on your overall health and well-being.

If you practice this juice diet correctly, you'll definitely get thinner and trimmer. Typical weight reduction varies from ½ pound to 1½ pounds (.23 to .68 kilograms) daily. But as with any other approach to weight loss, the big challenge is keeping the weight off once you start eating again. Fasting is not magic. If you revert to your pre-fast eating habits, you could easily put the weight back on. However, this 7-day juice diet, when repeated twice per year, has a proven track record for long-term weight reduction.

When you feel lighter, you're naturally motivated to sustain that good feeling. Your self-control improves, and bad habits fall away. And each time you repeat the 7-Day Just Juice Diet, the pounds you shed stay off for an increasingly longer period of time. It's neither a wonder pill nor a gimmicky promise. The diet works because you're retraining your system and reprogramming your body to have a new relationship with food.

In addition to cleaning you out, juices nourish you more thoroughly than solid foods. Your body digests, absorbs, and assimilates juice far more efficiently than it does solid food.

Weight loss, however desirable, is a bonus of this diet. The real purpose of these seven days is to detoxify. Your organs are subject to the accumulation of toxins that enter the body through food, water, and even the air. In addition, the body is naturally subject to toxins that are the byproducts of metabolism. The high-quality nutrients found in juices—phytochemical compounds, such as polyphenols—accelerate a chain reaction of detoxification that purges your organs of toxins that may have been stored there for years. Consider this an opportunity to pay some much-needed attention to your closest friends—your liver, gallbladder, kidneys, lungs, intestines, pancreas, and skin.

The Just Juice Diet is tremendously effective at helping to alleviate tough, persistent gastrointestinal problems. If you're bothered by inflammatory bowel disease, irritable bowel, leaky gut syndrome, colitis, constipation, or gluten intolerance, consider juice fasting. It's a wonderful way to rest the intestinal tissue and allow time for it to heal, rather than be continually irritated by the daily transit of food.

If you're suffering from allergies and food sensitivities, you owe it to yourself to try a juice fast. Fasting clears your system of the irritants in problematic foods and also heals the immune system. Fasting is like giving your immune system a makeover, allowing it to relax, recharge, and rebalance. If your body is unencumbered by stress and contaminants, your immune system will have a better chance of finding its natural balance, and the healing process will be more successful. Stabilizing, strengthening, and restoring balance to your immune system is a tall order, but fasting is arguably one of the easiest, most effective, and least expensive ways to do just that.

When you come off the fast, you'll have the opportunity to carefully reintroduce the foods that may give you problems and test whether you have a true sensitivity to them. This process will allow you to confirm whether you have specific food allergies or an out-of-whack immune system that will react to almost anything.

Skin rashes and conditions such as eczema are also helped by juice fasting, especially if you step up your exercise and increase your perspiration rate. Many skin ailments signal an underlying inflammation, intestinal irritation, imbalance in intestinal bacteria, or a combination of these. Skin problems are merely symptoms on the surface that mirror an internal disorder.

Finally, one of the great benefits of fasting on juice, or eating less in general, is feeling extra energy. (Conversely, one of the side effects of overeating is drowsiness!) Your body will be freed from most of the work of digestion, and you'll have access to all the energy that digestion would normally

Benefits of the 7-Day Just Juice Diet

A juice fast heals the immune system and cleanses major organs. It can also help to identify and relieve countless health conditions. The following are some of the benefits of the Just Juice Diet:

- blood purification
- colon cleansing
- hormone balance
- identification of food allergies
- improved gastrointestinal function
- improved nutrient assimilation
- liver detoxification
- relief from allergies

- relief from arthritis
- relief from chronic fatigue
- relief from eczema and other skin conditions
- relief from irritable bowel syndrome and colitis
- strengthened immune system
- weight loss

Take a Vacation from Supplements

These seven days of just juice provide a good opportunity to discontinue all nonessential supplements, including herbs, minerals, and vitamins. Sediment from these supplements can initiate the flow of digestive enzymes and stimulate a desire for food. Not what you want!

In addition, a vacation from supplements helps your body reestablish its natural biochemical balance. If you're constantly influencing your biochemistry by taking supplements, your system never has a chance to reset and return to a neutral place. Strangely enough, sometimes this small change can eliminate symptoms and health problems that all the supplements in the world couldn't resolve.

require. But if you want that extra energy to last, you must increase the efficiency of digestion and especially assimilation. That's because it's one thing to move food in and out—that's just plumbing. But it's another to deliver the nutrients in that food to your cells. The cleansing nature of this juice diet streamlines that process, just like cleaning your car's fuel injectors yields better gas mileage.

This juice diet is not likely to cure all of your health problems overnight. After all, one week does not reverse a lifetime of dietary imprudence. However, a week of just juice will help steer you back onto the right track.

CLEANSING WITH JUICE AND MORE

Your diet of fresh juices will be enhanced if you also employ cleansing techniques that tune up your internal organs (see chapter 5). Think of juices as cleansing solutions. The techniques you'll use to cleanse your internal organs act like a scrub brush, and all the liquids you consume while fasting rinse out contaminants.

During the week of the fast, you'll be spending lots of time in the kitchen juicing all that fabulous produce, but you should also expect to spend some quality time in the bathroom. This is, after all, a cleanse! Your goal will be to drink approximately one gallon (4 liters) of fluids every day. It's how you're going to flush your system.

Exercise also is an important part of this cleansing program. You don't want to overdo it, however, as you need to conserve your energy and allow your internal organs to perform the vital detoxification work you want and need. See pages 53 to 56 for appropriate exercises that enhance detoxification.

The five primary organs and systems that need detoxification are the intestines, lungs, liver, skin, and urinary tract. It's particularly important to focus on cleansing the organs that are essential for good digestion, the colon and the liver, and those of the urinary tract, the bladder and the kidneys.

Colon Cleansing

Colon-cleansing drinks are important elements in the Just Juice Diet. So plan to use one or more of the colon-cleanser recipes in this book (see pages 107 to 110); for a little additional help, you might want to use milk of magnesia (see sidebar, page 7). Certain therapies, such as colonics, also can enhance colon cleansing.

The colon-cleanser recipes are designed to keep a continuous supply of soluble fiber moving through the intestines. Soluble fiber dissolves in water and forms a gel or mucilage. It's not digestible; your stomach and pancreas will not respond to it with digestive secretions. However, you can expect to eventually pass this fiber as a bowel movement, which is positive proof that the fiber is working to remove toxins. Colon cleansers are gelatinous drinks that are not only excellent for cleansing, but they also can reduce appetite, alleviate constipation, soothe an irritable bowel, regulate blood sugar for diabetics, and lower cholesterol.

Psyllium seeds and flaxseeds are the primary sources of soluble fiber that you'll find in my recipes for colon-cleansing drinks. Psyllium seeds produce the greatest amount of gel per tablespoon, are very smooth, and have a neutral flavor. Flaxseeds produce half as much gel as psyllium seeds, are much more coarse, and have a delicious nutty flavor. Both are available in natural food stores; choose one or alternate between the two. You can buy flaxseeds that are already ground or you can make your own flaxseed powder if you have a blender that will pulverize them. (Interested in using chia instead? See page 47.)

The mucilage formed by these seeds is not only impervious to digestion, but it also envelopes all nutrients and prevents their absorption. For this reason, I recommend that you use only bottled, pasteurized juices for flavoring these drinks. You don't want to waste the precious nutrients in fresh juices by entrapping them in mucilage.

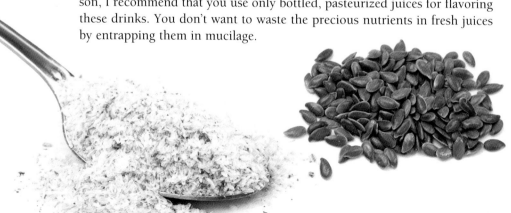

Milk of Magnesia

While the colon-cleansing drinks contain fibrous seeds that should keep things moving in your intestines, these drinks sometimes need a little help. That's the job of the laxative milk of magnesia, which is a natural, single-ingredient mineral product that was first sold in the early 1800s. Its chemical name is magnesium hydroxide, and despite the word "milk" in its name, it contains no dairy products. You can get milk of magnesia from any pharmacy, and it's cheap! Be sure to buy the plain stuff, without any coloring agents, sugar, or flavor additives.

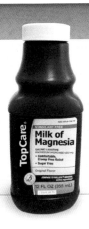

Liver Cleansing

The liver is an amazing organ with hundreds of functions relating to metabolism, including synthesizing nutrients; breaking down fats, drugs and other non-food substances; regulating cholesterol; storing glucose and vitamins; and much more. Some of those toxins are stored in the liver to prevent their general circulation. So the liver is arguably the most important organ for detoxification. Anything you do to relieve your liver of these toxic burdens improves its overall functioning and efficiency.

Although you can detoxify the liver with cleansing drinks, I also highly recommend massage and aerobic exercise to improve liver function. Although the liver is out of sight, it shouldn't be out of mind. Movement and flow are necessary to stimulate the liver to empty. See pages 60 to 63 for more information on additional therapies you can use to cleanse your liver.

Urinary Tract Cleansing

The urinary tract consists of the kidneys, the bladder, and the tubes (ureters) that connect them, along with the tube (urethra) that directs urine out of your body. In a way, the kidneys are inherently designed for detoxification because they continuously filter the blood and eliminate the waste products that human cells naturally produce. Urine is essentially freshly filtered liquid waste.

Like any filter, the kidneys need regular cleaning. Fasting is one of the best things you can do to rest, recharge, and cleanse your kidneys. Water fasting is even better than juice fasting, but in either case your kidneys get a break because they won't need to filter the immense load of waste products coming in from a normal diet. Plus, many of the juices you drink on the Just Juice Diet are naturally diuretic and aquaretic. (Diuretics increase the production of urine, and aquaretics increase urine flow without depleting electrolytes.) So not only do juices help you move water through your urinary tract, but they also help expel the waste the kidneys process. The juices of watermelon (including the rind), celery, parsley, wheatgrass, dandelion, cucumber, and garlic excel at flushing the kidneys.

Caring for your kidneys is critical for both your health and your pocketbook. A urologist will tell you that a used kidney goes for about $68,000. And that's not installed! So invest in keeping these filters running smoothly.

YOUR MIND-SET AND GOALS FOR THE JUICE FAST

Before you start assembling everything you need for the Just Juice Diet, take a moment to prepare yourself for the work you're about to do. Before you begin, it's important to ask yourself, "Why am I doing this?"

What are your goals? Is this your first time? Have you been wanting to do this for a long time? What kind of outcome do you want? Lose some weight? Stop frequent headaches? Decrease your overall toxic load? These goals are all legitimate, and they're all doable.

When you understand your motives for doing this juice diet, you'll find it easier to stay on the path when the road gets bumpy. Part of the prep work for fasting is getting in the right mind-set.

To this end, I recommend keeping a daily fasting diary (see page 51). Start by identifying your motives and goals and writing them down. Then keep track of what happens each day: what you drink, how you feel (both physically and mentally), and the times when you're up and the times when you're down. Documenting these details will give you a better understanding of where you are and where you've been, and you can use this information to determine if you need to make changes. For example, maybe you're not drinking enough or need to incorporate more cleansing drinks. Keeping a journal isn't a requirement, but it can help you distinguish the events and outcomes of one day from another and keep you on track.

Getting Ready for the Fast

Start to prepare yourself mentally and physically for the 7-Day Just Juice Fast.

- Set your mind to it.
- Clear your schedule (7 to 14 days).
- Order cleansing products (if necessary).
- Go food shopping.
- Make optional appointments for massage, bodywork, colonics, sauna, or steam bath.

Commit for One Week

Even though this diet is all about the body, you must get in the right frame of mind before you can begin. You may say, "Hey, Sproutman, I don't have the time for this stuff." But think of it this way. If you had to go to a health spa in the Caribbean, you'd make the time. You would focus 100 percent on your health. Unfortunately, some people are forced to do exactly this. They have to drop everything and travel to some faraway clinic because they let their health go. Don't let that happen to you.

Think of this week as a gift to yourself. You spend so much time taking care of your children, your spouse, your parents, your business, your car, your house . . . it's too easy to neglect yourself. Take better care of your body. This is your week to do that—a full week to devote to your body and your health. You'd take a vacation to relax and relieve stress. Think of this as an inner vacation.

Clear Your Schedule

One of the most important steps for planning a successful cleanse is to clear your schedule. You can continue to work at your job and maintain most of your regular routine. But for the best results, keep stressful events off your calendar for this week, plus a few days before and after. For example, try to schedule your fast to avoid birthdays, business lunches, trips, and parties. These events involve a smorgasbord of tasty foods that will only tempt you and force you into unnecessary discussions about why you aren't eating. During the week of your fast, give yourself a break from anything that typically drags you down. Allow yourself a little more private time and avoid distractions as much as possible.

You'll need a few days before the fast to get organized and three to four days afterward to come off the fast gradually. You may even find that you want to extend your cleanse a few days because you're on a roll! Allow a minimum of two weeks to do the juice diet right—or longer if you have bigger goals and are open to the possibility of extending your cleanse. You might also consider scheduling an appointment with your favorite bodyworker, getting a colonic, taking a sauna or steam bath, and doing daily aerobic exercise. These extras help promote deeper detoxification.

Evaluate the Risks

As long as you're not extremely ill or overweight, you should be able to successfully complete the 7-Day Just Juice Diet without medical supervision. In fact, you should come out of it better off than when you started. Typically, the

Should You Consult Your Doctor?

Consult with your doctor before starting the 7-Day Just Juice Diet if you're more than fifty pounds overweight, are taking medications for any reason, or if you have any of the following conditions:

- arrhythmia
- diabetes
- heart disease
- high blood pressure
- hypoglycemia

emotional side effects of not eating are more of a challenge than the physical effects. Taking a break from solid food for one week and doing some gentle cleansing is not considered life-threatening, and juice fasting is definitely not starving. In fact, the juices are super nourishing.

That said, everyone's situation is different. You won't be fasting in a clinic where you can be monitored, after all. If you have a health condition that you're concerned about, are more than fifty pounds overweight, or are taking medication for any reason, play it safe and consult your physician about your plan to do a juice fast. Although most doctors don't know much about fasting, your doctor should be aware of what you're doing and consent to your doing it. Your doctor may want to monitor you before, during, and after your fast. In addition, be sure to talk to your doctor about taking a break from medication. If you have diabetes, you may want to discuss reducing your insulin dosage according to your daily numbers.

Conditions such as diabetes, high blood pressure, and hypoglycemia can be helped by fasting. If you have one or more of these conditions, your body may be particularly sensitive to changes in diet, and your fast may involve a few ups and downs. Choosing to use medications or juice fasting to control these conditions is like choosing between driving on a straight and level turnpike or taking a mountain road. You'll reach your destination in either case, but you may need some professional assistance to help you handle the curves.

Flock Together

We live in a food-oriented culture, so people are likely to show their surprise when you announce your intentions to go on a juice fast: "What? You're not eating for a week?!" Be prepared for some flak. Your family may not understand you, and your friends may think you're weird. You've got three choices: keep to yourself as much as possible, find a partner to do this with, or surround yourself with a community of like-minded people.

In my experience, the folks who are most successful with juice fasting join a group, participating either in person or online. Getting the support of a group, plus the guidance of a coach, is an ideal way to juice fast. And thanks to the Internet, it's now possible to join a juice-fasting group no matter where you live. I hope one day you can join me online for one of my Just Juice webinars. See resources, page 127, for more information.

WHAT YOU CAN EXPECT DURING A JUICE FAST

Once you get going, spending a week to clean out and lighten up is easier than you think. For most people, juice fasting is smooth sailing much of the time. I can promise that you won't starve, and you'll feel like you have more energy than usual. But there *is* a cycle. Your energy level will go up and down, just like it does when you're not fasting.

The Challenge of the First Three Days

Once you start fasting, it takes about three days for your digestive organs to relax their daily production of enzymes. The secretion of these enzymes is part of the natural cycle that creates feelings of hunger. So with each passing day, your desire for food will diminish as the enzyme flow decreases. No secretions means no hunger. However, even small food particles can prompt enzyme production, so during this time, it's important to strain your juices to remove any fiber or other sediment. If you drink only strained liquids, your enzyme secretions will cease—and so will your desire for food. Because eating is so habitual, these first two to three days will require some self-control. Expect this challenge, prepare for it, and you'll easily get beyond it.

If you've never fasted before, you can imagine that it might be a shock to your system to suddenly stop eating. That's why I've designed a structured program that includes a pre-fasting diet as well as a transition period that eases you back into eating solid foods. You can expect the first three days of the fast to be an adjustment period, but it's nothing you can't handle. Remember your original motivation and intentions, and hold on to your determination.

The Healing Crisis

During the fast, you may experience something called a "healing crisis." If so, you may actually feel worse for a little while instead of better. Cleansing involves the movement of toxins through your bloodstream and food material

Ask Sproutman

Dear Sproutman: I started my juice fast yesterday. I have a headache, a bit of nausea, some aches, and a fever. Any thoughts on how to tell the difference between a healing reaction and a real flu? —*Susan*

Dear Susan: The symptoms can be similar, but since you just started fasting yesterday, you haven't detoxed enough yet to generate these reactions. Only fasts of ten days or longer are capable of kicking in an immune response as dramatic as a fever (which, by the way, is part of your body's natural cleansing process). Therefore, you most likely have the flu.

through your intestines. If you're getting rid of more toxins than your body would normally handle, you might experience headaches, nausea, fatigue, irritability, anxiety, depression, or a decrease in your ability to concentrate. One of the more acute symptoms of detoxification is fever. While temporarily uncomfortable, these experiences aren't bad news. Rather, they're signs that your body is in an elimination phase. Shake those toxins loose!

The goal of the Just Juice Diet in the first place is to shake toxins out of your body and eliminate them. (In fact, if you're not experiencing any symptoms of a healing crisis, you might not be doing enough to generate results.) Think of fasting as an adventure. If you were to go white-water rafting, you would fully expect to get wet, even a little roughed up and shaken. That's part of the process. The same is true for fasting. The more faithfully you follow the Just Juice Diet, the more toxins you'll eliminate, and the going might be rough some of the time. Fortunately, there are practices that can mitigate uncomfortable reactions by enhancing the exit of toxins, and you'll learn more about these in chapter 5.

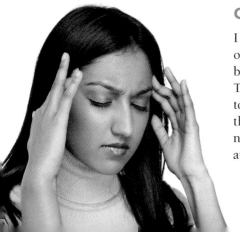

Can You Still Have Your Daily Coffee?

I recommend that you consider going off coffee and other heavily caffeinated drinks during the juice fast, because abstinence will allow for a deeper cleanse. The best approach is to quit gradually, starting one to two days prior to beginning the fast. You could thin your coffee with hot water, cut back on the number of cups per day, drink smaller amounts at a time, or switch to decaf coffee. (Decaf has only

Kicking the Coffee Habit

If you're a coffee drinker, you have a decision to make during the juice fast: drink it or drop it. Consider the following pros and cons:

The upside of kicking your habit:

- A fast cleanses your body and restarts your system, so now may be the perfect time to stop drinking coffee or make other dietary changes.
- It's always beneficial to take a break from something you do habitually—even something that's good for you, such as taking vitamins.

The downside of kicking your habit:

- If you abruptly stop drinking coffee, you're likely to have a headache and possibly other withdrawal symptoms that can last for days.
- Coffee withdrawal can produce symptoms similar to any addiction withdrawal—fatigue, drowsiness, irritability, and decreased concentration.

about 20 percent of the caffeine of regular coffee.) You could also substitute with green tea or other healthy, lightly caffeinated drinks. It's best to start this process prior to beginning the fast. Solid food helps mitigate the effects of withdrawal, even if it just serves as an emotional crutch.

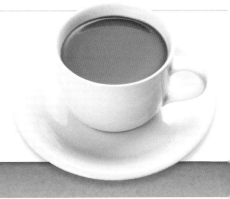

Still Craving the Caffeine?

If you do experience caffeine withdrawal, the most bothersome symptom is likely to be a persistent headache. To treat it, try the following techniques:

- Take a nap.
- Drink a lot of water.
- Suck on peppermints.
- Get an acupuncture treatment.
- Go for a colonic.

- Do aerobic exercise.
- Practice gentle yoga poses (no inversions or forward bends).
- Use plain aspirin sparingly (see below).

While I don't recommend becoming dependent on aspirin, you may feel the need to take it. Plain aspirin, without additives, is simply salicylic acid, a natural substance that was originally synthesized from the bark of the willow tree. Judicious use of plain aspirin may be all you need to get through tough times.

The goal is to make the transition less dramatic and therefore more tolerable. Tapering off the amount of caffeine you consume will decrease the intensity of your side effects and enable you to better cope with the withdrawal process. One more point: if you opt for an alternative hot drink during the fast, don't add milk or sweetener of any kind.

CAN'T MAINTAIN THE JUICE DIET?
TRY A SMOOTHIE INSTEAD.

Although most people manage the Just Juice Diet without problems, others may find along the way that they're not prepared for it, it's just the wrong time, or it's too much to manage. If you're not sure you can follow through, I encourage you to remember the reasons you chose to do this. However, if you feel you're truly in over your head, you do have an out. You can switch to using your blender instead of your juicer, which essentially means switching to a smoothie cleanse instead of doing a juice fast. This involves processing whole fruits and mostly green vegetables into smoothies for the week. Although the results won't be as dramatic or quick as those achieved during a juice fast, drinking fruit and vegetable smoothies is still very cleansing.

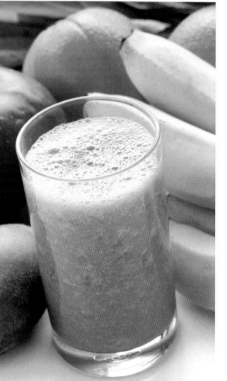

Let's be clear, though: drinking smoothies is not a fast. Because you're consuming liquified whole foods, not juices, your digestive system is working almost as much as it would if you were eating. The blender is simply doing the chewing for you. You won't get as great a benefit from a smoothie cleanse as you would from a juice fast, and this book is not a guide for a smoothie cleanse. Still, smoothies are a good option for cleansing, and if a smoothie cleanse is a better fit for you, by all means consider it. (Check out my Green Smoothie Online Cleanses in the resources listed on page 127.)

Learn more about the Green Smoothie Cleanse at
7DayJustJuiceDiet.com.

2

Getting Started with the 7-Day Just Juice Diet

Your food intake on the Just Juice Diet will be quite extensive—it's just going to be all liquid. You won't be bored with this liquid diet, I promise. In fact, you'll be very busy and possibly quite full, striving to drink 1 gallon (4 quarts or 4 liters) of fluids daily.

You'll drink 1 quart (liter) of four different kinds of liquids each day. The four equal parts are easy to remember. The first quart is pure water. Second comes vegetable juice (pages 17 to 19): you'll drink at least 1 quart of fresh green vegetable juice, which will be the core of your therapy. The more green juice you drink, the deeper the cleansing and the more detoxification you'll likely experience. The third quart of liquid is colon cleansers, and I provide recipes for these on pages 107 to 110.

The fourth and final quart is made up of several different drinks, including liver cleansers and sweet juice, made fresh from sweet vegetables, fruits, or both. In addition, you can choose from fresh-squeezed citrus or pineapple juice, herbal tea, hot vegetable broth, or anything from the list of optional drinks (see page 22).

In this chapter I'll give you my recommendations for the best vegetables and fruits to use for juicing. You'll find detailed information about the juicing process itself in chapter 3.

One more thing. Your cleanse will be more successful if you incorporate probiotic supplements every day. For more information, see page 24.

PURE WATER

Water is fundamental to cleansing. In fact, ancient healing traditions included fasting that was done only with water. While water fasting

The Just Juice Diet in a Nutshell

Here's a breakdown of what you'll drink each day:

- pure water, 1 quart (1 liter), within 20 minutes for the Water Flush
- fresh green vegetable juices, 1 quart (1 liter)
- colon cleansers, 1 quart (1 liter)
- other drinks totaling 1 quart (1 liter) or more, including:
  - liver cleanser, 8 to 16 ounces (250 to 500 ml)
  - sweet juice, no more than 16 ounces (500 ml)
  - your choice of fresh citrus juice, herbal tea, green juice from powder, and other optional drinks

effectively promotes detoxification and healing, juice fasting does so while providing all your body systems with exceptional nutrition.

The Water Flush

The Water Flush is something you'll do each morning, and it requires you to drink 1 quart (1 liter) of pure water in 20 minutes. Consuming this much water in such a short period of time overwhelms the capacity of the urinary tract, forcing much of the water to reroute to the intestinal tract instead. If you do this successfully, you'll be moving your bowels within

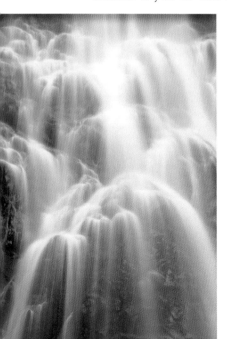

1 hour of drinking the full amount of water. It's best to do this on an empty stomach and preferably first thing in the morning; that way you'll have less material to empty out. Room temperature water is recommended. Cold water will cause your digestive system to contract, and hot water will be difficult to consume quickly.

The Water Flush is easy for some people and difficult for others. Why? Because it involves a certain degree of guzzling! If you don't get a response after drinking 1 quart (1 liter) of water in 20 minutes, try increasing the volume or decreasing the time it takes to drink. You might also increase the amount of milk of magnesia you take before bedtime or take an extra 1 to 2 tablespoons (15 to 30 milliliters) in the morning before you start drinking.

This top-down flush is part of your daily practice on this cleanse. If you're having difficulty with it, you can certainly skip a day, but generally most people find it doable, simple, and effective. The Water Flush is a less-demanding alternative to enemas and colonics, which a lot of people appreciate. It's not a direct replacement, but it provides some of the same benefits.

Clean Water

During the 7-Day Just Juice Diet, drink the purest water you can find. That recommendation inevitably leads to the big question: which water is best? That's not always easy to determine.

Buying water and schlepping it home is inconvenient, time consuming, and expensive. And we don't need any more plastic! In my book *Water, the Ultimate Cure,* I compare various water-purifying devices, such as reverse osmosis units, distillers, carbon blocks, and ultraviolet and ozone purifiers. All have their advantages and disadvantages. The purifying device you select must be up to the task of treating the specific pollutants in your drinking water, whether you get it from a municipal system or a country well. Your goal is to get the cleanest water possible. And drink at least 1 quart of it every day of the juice fast.

FRESH GREEN VEGETABLE JUICES

Y ou'll be drinking 1 full quart of fresh vegetable juice each day, so be prepared to make a few batches. My green vegetable juice recipes (see pages 97 to 104) incorporate lots of crucifers, such as broccoli, cabbage, collards, and kale. These vegetables are highly therapeutic, and you can choose your favorites. You may prefer to stick with what's easiest, and that's fine. Juicing cabbage is a lot more work than juicing kale or collard greens, for example, because you have to cut it into pieces to feed it through the chute of your juicer. Collard or kale leaves are a natural fit for juicers, because they're long and slender. You can make juicing kale even easier by choosing lacinato or Russian kale, because the leaves of these varieties are straighter and flatter than those of common curly kale.

Carrots, celery, cucumbers, and parsley also fit conveniently inside a feed chute. When you buy carrots, try to get skinny ones that will fit through the chute without being cut. Leafy parsley is also easy to juice. The juicer accepts it quickly, practically stealing it from your hand. I'm not suggesting you limit yourself to juicing only long, narrow vegetables. Indeed, I encourage you to use a variety. Beets, for example, may require a little more prep work, but they're worth it.

Along with crucifers, a vegetable that is wonderful to add to your fresh juice is spinach. I realize that some people are concerned about the oxalic

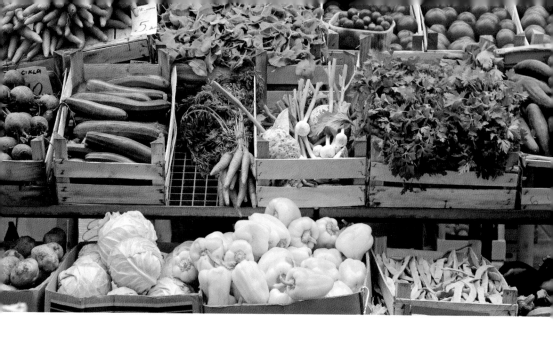

acid found in spinach. This compound can potentially combine with calcium to form calcium oxalate—the stuff that makes kidney stones. Spinach may have a reputation for having a lot of oxalic acid, but this compound is found in all sorts of vegetables, nuts, beans, grains, breads, berries, meats, dairy products, and even chocolate. Kidney specialists agree that as long as you don't have kidney problems, your body is fully capable of managing oxalic acid, even in the larger amounts you might consume by juicing. So drink your spinach with peace of mind and enjoy its rich nutrition.

One alternative to fresh green vegetable juice is a drink made from green juice powder. If you're having a busy day or following the Lite Plan (see page 42), you can make a green juice from a high-quality green juice powder (see page 23). Drinks made from green juice powder can be enjoyed anytime.

RECOMMENDED VEGETABLES FOR JUICING

As you prepare for the 7-Day Just Juice Diet, one of your first concerns will be learning what vegetables are best for juicing. The following is a general list of the vegetables you can juice; choosing organic should be a priority:

- alfalfa sprouts
- beets
- bell peppers (green or red)
- broccoli
- Brussels sprouts
- cabbage

- carrots
- celery
- collards
- cucumbers
- garlic

- ginger
- kale
- parsley
- spinach
- tomatoes

You don't need to purchase or use all the items on this list. Keep it simple. Some juice recipes include only three or four ingredients. Check out my combinations in the recipes on pages 97 to 104.

COLON-CLEANSING DRINKS

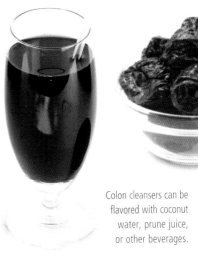

This juice fast is all about cleansing, and that's why each day you'll drink one quart of colon-cleansing drinks and a liver-cleansing drink to boot. Now, cleansing drinks, or "cleansers" as I call them, may not sound appetizing, and they may even seem a bit mysterious and complicated. But rest assured, these drinks are made from a few simple ingredients and require even less fuss than juicing.

Colon cleansers can be flavored with coconut water, prune juice, or other beverages.

Colon cleansers are made primarily from seeds (flaxseeds or psyllium seeds) and commercial beverages, such as coconut water, prune juice, or unsweetened nondairy milks (such as almond milk). This is the stuff that keeps things moving along. See my recipes on pages 107 to 110.

LIVER-CLEANSING DRINKS

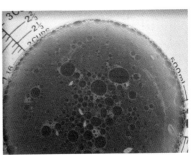

Liver cleansers include juices made from grapefruit, lemon, and wheatgrass, as well as hot lemon tea and a beverage made from apple cider vinegar. See the recipes on pages 111 and 113. Be sure to include 8 to 16 ounces (250 to 500 milliliters) of the Grapefruit Liver Cleanser recipe (page 111) in your regimen every day.

Spots of olive oil in Grapefruit Liver Cleanser.

Ask Sproutman

Dear Sproutman: What's the purpose of the olive oil in the Grapefruit Liver Cleanser (page 111)? —*Judith*

Dear Judith: A small amount of olive oil actually stimulates the gallbladder to secrete bile. Much more oil than this would force the gallbladder to process it, but a small amount merely wakes up the gland. It responds by releasing bile, which is a cleansing action.

OTHER DRINKS

If variety is the spice of life, then the Just Juice Diet has plenty of spice. From fresh fruit juices to bottled drinks (such as kombucha) and green juices mixed from powder, there's plenty to choose from. You can drink another quart daily from the following suggestions in this "other drinks" category.

SWEET JUICES AND FRUIT JUICES

My sweet juice recipes (see pages 105 and 106) include fruits as well as some of the sweeter vegetables, such as beets. Fruits are secondary to vegetables in this cleanse because they contain more sugar, which should not be prevalent in this diet. Sugar sets up a whole metabolic process that's counterproductive to detoxification. Overindulging in sugar contributes to obesity, diabetes, parasites, autoimmune problems, and even cancer. While fruit is a lot better than soda or candy bars, the sugar in fruit still stimulates the growth of pathogens. And if you feed your pathogens high-quality, natural organic sugar, they'll love you even more!

I recommend that you limit the amount of sweet juice you drink during the fast. Sweet juices, as the name makes abundantly clear, are made from sweet fruits (apples, grapes, oranges, and watermelon) and sweet vegetables (beets and carrots). Restrict your daily intake of these drinks to about 16 ounces (500 milliliters) per day. If you have a health condition that is worsened by sugar, such as candida or diabetes, restrict your consumption of sweet juice even more.

You need not be concerned about the quantity of fresh juice you drink when it's obtained from less sugary fruits, such as citrus and pineapple. Citrus fruits, including grapefruits, lemons, and limes, are in a special class.

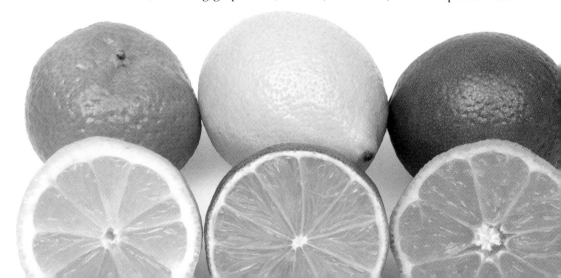

These fruits are natural cleansers, and you can drink fresh citrus juices daily. They contain considerable amounts of limonene, a natural solvent found in the rind and pulp. Limonene is capable of dissolving gallstones, which is why citrus fruits are part of your daily Grapefruit Liver Cleanser (page 111). Limonene also fights the onset and growth of cancer. Grapefruit seeds, pulp, and membranes contain a compound called GSE, or grapefruit seed extract. GSE is antimicrobial and has been used effectively in the treatment of candidiasis and other harmful yeast and bacterial infections.

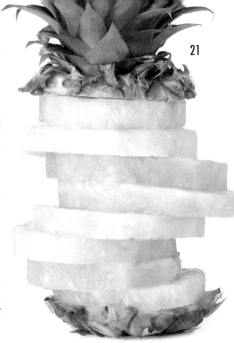

Pineapple is another strong natural cleanser, and on this cleanse pineapple juice can be consumed regularly. Pineapple is one of the best sources of bromelain, an enzyme that breaks down protein, reduces inflammation, and serves as an anticancer agent.

By the way, not all fruits are juiceable. Bananas, cantaloupes, and mangoes won't release their juice. For example, put a banana through your juicer, and you'll notice it all comes out the pulp ejector. No juice is extracted! These fruits work best in smoothies, which are made in a blender and allow you to consume the fruit with all its fiber. However, that's not what you want to be doing this week, when the emphasis is on cleansing and detoxification.

Recommended Fruits for Juicing

The fresh-squeezed juices I recommend for the Just Juice Diet include the following fruits; choosing organic should be a priority:

- apples
- grapes
- grapefruit
- lemons
- limes
- oranges
- pineapple
- watermelon

Stock up on plenty of these items as you begin the Just Juice Diet and get ready to give not only your juicer but also your citrus juicer a weeklong workout. See pages 105 to 106 for sweet juice recipes.

Ask Sproutman

Dear Sproutman: You say "go light on the sweets," but beets and carrots are included on your veggie list, and they're sweet. So how much or how little carrot should I be including in my drinks? —*Rob*

Dear Rob: Some vegetable juices aren't really sweet. For example, when you mix carrots with veggies that aren't sweet, the overall sweetness of the drink is reduced. For instance, combining carrots with celery and cucumbers results in a juice that's not sweet—so you can drink more of it. However, you can make very sweet juices by mixing carrots with other sweet veggies, such as beets, and sweet fruits, such as apples. Limit drinks like these to about 16 ounces (500 milliliters) per day during the juice fast. Sweet juices are a great pick-me-up, but they're not as therapeutic as vegetable juices. Think of them as a dessert and enjoy them as a treat—but don't make them the foundation of the Just Juice Diet.

OPTIONAL DRINKS

Although fresh vegetable and fruit juices are the core of this diet and necessary for optimum success, there are lots of other things you can drink that don't require you to use (or clean) your juicer or visit the juice bar. For example, grab a coconut water or a bottled drink at the natural food store. Here's a list of some of the optional drinks you can choose:

- aloe vera juice
- Apple Cider Vinegar Drink (page 112)
- vegetable or miso broths, hot (strained)
- coconut water
- green juice from powder (see page 23)

- herbal teas (see page 23)
- kombucha
- nondairy milk (plain, unsweetened)
- noni juice
- pickle juice, raw
- sauerkraut juice, raw

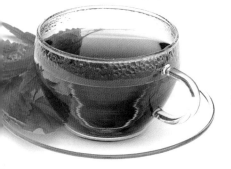

During this fast, when you're not eating cooked food, you may crave some heat in liquid form. Need a steaming mug of wholesome goodness to warm you up? Hot vegetable or miso broths (see recipes, pages 115 to 117) or hot herbal teas, such as those in the following list, are welcome options.

- chamomile
- cinnamon
- dandelion
- fennel
- ginger (page 114)
- ginseng

- lemon (page 113)
- licorice
- mint
- red clover
- your favorite brand of detox tea

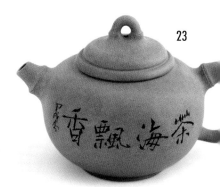

GREEN JUICE FROM POWDER

While the emphasis during this cleanse is on freshly juiced green vegetables, I also recommend green juice from powder. Green juice powder typically is made from wheatgrass juice or juices from wheatgrass and other grasses, such as barley grass. Green juice is an optional drink you can use to add convenience to your cleanse. See resources, page 127, for the green juice powders I recommend.

Grass, of course, is what cows and horses graze on all day, and the juice from that grass has been sustaining their large, muscular bodies for thousands of generations. Although we now have research on the healing properties of grass, we need only look at these animals to conclude that it must be super-nutritious. Unlike cows, we can't digest grass, but we can drink grass juice, especially wheatgrass juice. Juice bars everywhere serve wheatgrass juice, or you can grow your own wheatgrass and juice it at home.

Aside from juice bars, the alternative to growing and juicing your own wheatgrass is to buy the juice in either frozen or powdered form. Frozen wheatgrass juice is sold in natural food stores, and so is the powdered variety. Powdered wheatgrass juice is particularly convenient to use because you can quickly turn the powder into a drink without using a juicer. But you must use a high-quality wheatgrass juice powder. The key words here are "juice powder." Wheatgrass juice powder is the dried solids from evaporated wheatgrass juice. It literally melts in your mouth. This is *not* the same as whole wheatgrass that's simply been dried and powdered. Powdered wheatgrass is the whole plant; juice powder is the whole plant juiced and the juice dehydrated. On the Just Juice Diet, you just need juice! And high-quality wheatgrass juice powder will be both convenient and super nutritious. Just make sure you're purchasing the right product.

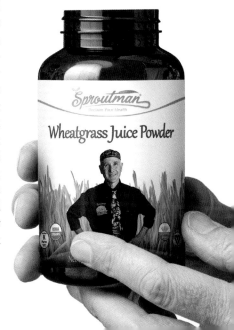

Wheatgrass juice powder is actually more nutritious than fresh wheat-grass juice because it's twenty-five times more concentrated. It takes about 25 pounds (11 kilograms) of fresh grass to yield 1 pound (450 grams) of evaporated grass juice powder. Of course, the process of evaporating the juice must be completed in the absence of heat and without exposure to oxygen, otherwise the newly exposed and fragile nutrients would degrade. This is why you must pick your brands carefully.

7DayJustJuiceDiet.com

There are lots of comparisons to be made between the different forms of wheatgrass—fresh, frozen, and powdered. Each has its pros and cons. You can find more discussion and comparisons in my book *Wheatgrass: Nature's Finest Medicine*.

Ask Sproutman

Dear Sproutman: I just bought some kombucha and was surprised to read that it's made in a base with sugar. —*Kurt*

Dear Kurt: Unfortunately, sugar is necessary as a base for the kombucha culture to grow on. In this sense, the sugar is a prebiotic. Although I'm opposed to using sugar in general, the probiotic activity of the culture and other healthful nutrients in kombucha help counter the effects of the sugar, making kombucha a good option during a juice fast. That is not the case with soft drinks!

PROBIOTICS IN THE JUST JUICE DIET

There are trillions of beneficial bacteria lining the walls of your intestines. These organisms are part of what's called your "microbiome"—all the microorganisms living inside you that influence your health in ways that scientists are now just beginning to fully appreciate. These microorganisms help keep the growth of harmful bacteria at bay. They also increase the absorption of nutrients, break down fats and sugar, and fight cancer cells. Bowel disease and food sensitivities are often a result of bacterial imbalances in the intestinal tract. In fact, scientists are starting to associate illnesses that you wouldn't think have any relationship to digestion, such as allergies, arthritis, asthma, and skin problems, with a lack of beneficial bacteria.

Problems occur when the delicate balance between good and bad bacteria goes out of whack. This balance can be disrupted by a bad diet, but the biggest culprit is antibiotics. They kill both good and bad bacteria. One important goal of cleansing is to reduce the population of unfriendly bacteria and replace it with helpful bacteria.

One way to reset this balance is to eat fermented foods, such as sauerkraut, yogurt, miso, tempeh, pickles, or kimchee, which are naturally rich in good bacteria. Another way to encourage the growth of good bacteria is to take probiotic supplements. Of course, during a juice fast, the only option is to use high-quality supplements because you're not eating solid foods. These supplements are highly concentrated, containing billions of beneficial bacteria per serving.

I recommend daily probiotic supplementation of up to 50 billion friendly bacteria, such as lactobacillus and bifidobacteria, during the Just Juice Diet. Probiotics can affect your bowel movements, increasing output, so introduce them gradually. Start with half the recommended dose (about 25 billion friendly bacteria per day) for the first two days, then build up to taking the full amount. When you can, take half of your daily probiotics in the morning and half in the evening, but avoid taking them at the same time as a colon cleanser or hot drink. For more information about when to take probiotics, see the sidebar, page 50.

Probiotics are an essential part of this program, and because probiotics are living bacteria, it's essential to choose high-quality supplements. See the resources (page 126) for brands I recommend.

ORGANICS ARE A PRIORITY

Make every effort to buy organic fruits and vegetables for your juice fast. The introduction of agricultural chemicals into our food chain, groundwater, air, and soil has had a devastating and insidious effect on public health. There's a lot of evidence that these chemicals are some of the most potent cancer-causing substances ever produced. For this reason, buying organic food should always be a priority. During this week of fasting, it's especially important to go organic. This is a cleanse, after all, and your intention is to get rid of toxins, not add them by juicing contaminated fruits and vegetables.

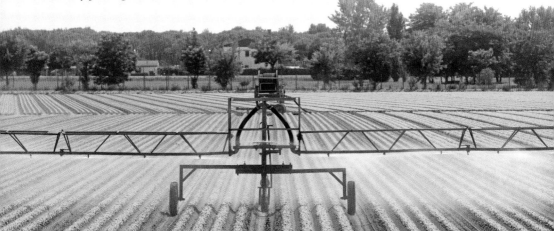

When you're at the produce stand, you have many decisions to make, and price is always a factor. Organic produce is usually more expensive than conventionally grown fruits and vegetables, but are you really saving money by not eating the cleanest food you can find? Why risk ingesting even small doses of artificial fertilizers, fumigants, insecticides, and herbicides? The cost of being ill is so astronomical that medical bills cause 62 percent of the bankruptcies in America according to a study published in the *American Journal of Medicine* in 2012. Compare bankruptcy to the few pennies per pound that organic produce costs over conventional fruits and vegetables, and I think you'll see that purchasing organic is indubitably a good investment for your health.

Some fruits and vegetables are more contaminated by chemicals than others. See the sidebar, page 85, for a list.

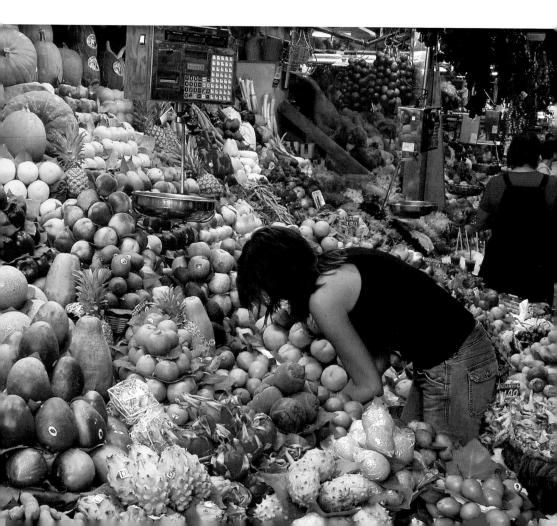

Your Juice Diet Shopping Lists

The following lists contain the ingredients you'll need for the fast, but you don't need to buy all the fresh produce at once. Start with the suggested quantities; as you go along, you'll get a better feel for how much you need and what you like best. Besides, you can only fit so much in your refrigerator!

VEGETABLES

Vegetables, including leafy greens, are the stars of the Just Juice Diet and the fresh green vegetable juices. The quantities suggested here may last you only one or two days, but you can always buy more:

- 2 bunches kale
- 1 bunch celery
- 1 bunch parsley
- 4 lemons
- 1 garlic bulb
- 2-inch piece fresh ginger

FRUITS

Fresh fruits are necessary for the sweet juice recipes. If you prefer not to drink sweet juice, you'll still need the lemons and grapefruits, which are essential for the Grapefruit Liver Cleanser:

- 4 grapefruits
- 4 lemons
- 4 apples
- 1 pound (450 grams) carrots
- 1 pound (450 grams) beets (3 medium)
- 1 pineapple

INGREDIENTS FOR CLEANSING DRINKS

- flaxseeds or psyllium seeds, finely ground
- prune juice or coconut water
- plain unsweetened nondairy milk
- olive oil, small bottle
- liquid bentonite clay (optional)

OTHER CLEANSING SUPPLIES

- milk of magnesia (any brand without coloring agents, sugar, and flavor additives) or RenewLife CleanseMore (see resources, page 125)
- probiotics (see resources, page 126)
- activated charcoal tablets (optional)
- 2-quart (2-liter) enema bag (optional)
- Epsom salts (allow up to 3 pounds or 1.5 kilograms per bath)

OTHER DRINKS

Select from the variety of optional drinks and teas (see page 22) and green juice powder (see resources, page 127).

TABLE 1. Juice volume from common fruits and vegetables

FRUIT OR VEGETABLE	SIZE, QUANTITY, OR WEIGHT	VOLUME OF JUICE
Apple, Granny Smith	1 (2.5 inches/6 centimeters)	5 ounces (165 milliliters)
Beets	3 medium (1 pound/450 grams)	6 ounces (185 milliliters)
Bell pepper	1 (8 ounces/225 grams)	6 ounces (185 milliliters)
Carrots	1 pound	8 ounces (250 milliliters)
Carrots	10 (7 inches/18 centimeters)	13 ounces (410 milliliters)
Celery	7 stalks	14 ounces (440 milliliters)
Collard leaves	10 leaves (9 ounces/255 grams)	8 ounces (250 milliliters)
Dill, fresh	4 ounces (115 grams)	2 ounces (60 milliliters)
Gingerroot	1 inch (2.5 centimeters)	0.25 ounces (1 tablespoon/ 15 milliliters)
Grapefruit	1 (3.5 inches/9 centimeters)	6 to 8 ounces (185 to 250 milliliters)
Kale, lacinato	15 stalks	6 ounces (185 milliliters)
Kale, baby	5 ounces (140 grams)	4 ounces (125 milliliters)
Lemon	1	2 ounces (60 milliliters)
Parsley	10 large sprigs	1 ounce (30 milliliters)
Spinach, savoy	12 ounces (340 grams)	7 ounces (220 milliliters)
Tomato	1 (3 inches/8 centimeters)	8 to 9 ounces (250 to 280 milliliters)
Wheatgrass	8 ounces (225 grams)	5 ounces (165 milliliters)

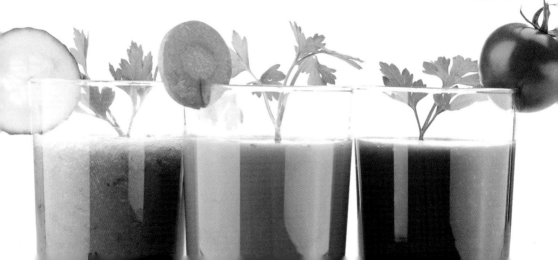

3

Selecting the Right Juicer and Juicing Efficiently

Knowing how to select a juicer, use a juicer, and make good juice is central to the Just Juice Diet. Happily, I report that none of this is difficult to learn. If you start with high-quality equipment, making juice is about as easy as assembling a fresh salad: just prepare the produce and decide what combinations you'd like to try. Let me give you some advice on selecting a juicer, then I'll walk you through how to use it efficiently.

WHICH JUICER IS BEST?

When it comes to producing nutritious results, a fruit and vegetable juicer is without question the most important appliance in your home. The juices you'll consume are so rich in vitamins and minerals, they could replace hundreds of dollars' worth of supplements. And that doesn't take into account all the fun you and your family will have using this appliance. A juicer is a fountain-of-youth machine that conjures up flavors and colors potent enough to seduce even the most soda-addicted family member.

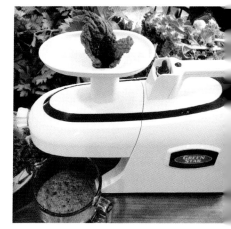

All juicers are not equal. They've become so popular that you can find a wide range, in terms of both price and quality. Inexpensive machines can go for US$99, whereas machines with special presses and stainless steel casings might cost up to US$1,000. But most quality juicers cost between

$300 and $600, and the good ones will last a lifetime. Buy from a manufacturer that specializes in juicers and has a solid reputation for quality. Just be aware that manufacturers make a dizzying array of claims as to why their particular juicers are superior to others.

Whatever juicer you choose, the most important question is this: will you use it? Choose a machine that is convenient to use and that you'll be happy to work with on a daily basis. Here are some of the features you should understand, so you can choose a juicer that best suits your needs.

A juicer is a fountain-of-youth machine that conjures up flavors and colors potent enough to seduce even the most soda-addicted family member.

Extraction

The two types of juicers are centrifugal and masticating, and these machines extract juice differently. Centrifugal juicers slice the vegetables with sharp blades that spin at 3,000 to 13,000 RPMs. Not only does that speed create short-term friction and damaging heat, but the blades also move so quickly they can never get deep into the cell walls of the vegetables or fruit. Slow masticating juicers, on the other hand, triturate, or "chew," the produce you're juicing and break open cell walls, releasing more nutrients. Masticating juicers grind and squeeze, while centrifugal juicers quickly slice and spin.

Speed

Faster is not always better. There's nothing to be gained from processing juice rapidly—speed causes oxidation and friction, leading to heat that destroys nutrients. If you see a juicer that measures its speed in the thousands of RPMs, walk away. The best juicers revolve at less than 100 RPMs, and some go as low as 47 RPMs (the equivalent of cranking a hand juicer). The slower a juicer's speed, the more nutrients it preserves during processing. Slow-speed machines work well for juicing wheatgrass too.

I describe slow machines as "therapeutic" juicers, because they dig deeper into plant tissues and extract more phytonutrients. Therapeutic juicers are generally worm-gear machines.

In these juicers, the gear looks like a big screw that slowly squeezes produce into pulp. Inexpensive

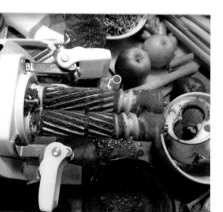
Twin stainless steel gears hard at work.

slow juicers have a single plastic gear, or auger. Higher-priced machines use two side-by-side gears that are made of stainless steel. These twin-gear machines are generally considered the best in the industry. Even better are machines that include magnets and ceramics inside the twin-auger gears. They create a magnetic field that influences the water molecules in the juice as it passes through. Although it may sound like hocus-pocus, this process is actually grounded in good science. As the water molecules straighten, the stability of the juice increases. As evidence, you can actually taste the difference. Moreover, fresh juice survives much longer in the refrigerator when it's been made under the influence of magnets.

Although the standard advice for years has been "juice and drink immediately," it's not always practical to follow this old axiom. Increasing the stability and longevity of your juice can make the process of juicing more efficient and convenient. The prospect of juicing once every day or two versus multiple times daily is certainly appealing to many people. (See "Storing and Transporting Fresh Juice," page 36.)

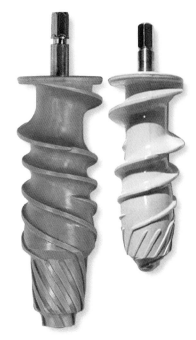

Two single-auger plastic gears from different manufacturers. Shorter means they're in contact with the vegetables for less time.

All single- and twin-gear machines include pulp ejectors. These ejectors allow you to juice continuously without stopping to clean out a basketful of pulp. This is a handy feature; if you wanted, you could make a full gallon of juice at once without ever stopping to clean out the pulp.

Convenience

When it comes to using a juicer, convenience of operation and ease of clean-up are very important factors. If you're discouraged by how difficult it is to set up and clean your juicer, you'll probably use it less frequently. An unused juicer does nothing for your health.

Citrus Juicers

For making citrus juice, such as my Grapefruit Liver Cleanser (page 111), a common electric citrus juicer is your best option. It's convenient, fast, and affordable. Although single-auger juicers do make a creamy citrus juice, they require a lot more time peeling and inserting the fruit.

Ask Sproutman

Dear Sproutman: Can you juice the skin of lemon or grapefruit? —*Carolyn*

Dear Carolyn: The flavor of citrus skins is very strong and can overpower an otherwise delicious juice. If you want to try juicing citrus skin, use only a small amount. After all, the limonene extracted from lemon skin is potent enough to dissolve gallstones! That's why it's such a powerful cleansing agent.

All juicers have a cutter blade, or gear; a cover; a screen; and a housing, or juicer body; all of these parts must be removed and cleaned after each use. Sure, there are differences among various machines, but in the end, how quick and easy it is to clean a particular juicer is a matter of practice —the more you do it, the easier it will become and the more efficient you will get.

If you're discouraged by how difficult it is to set up and clean your juicer, you'll probably use it less frequently. An unused juicer does nothing for your health.

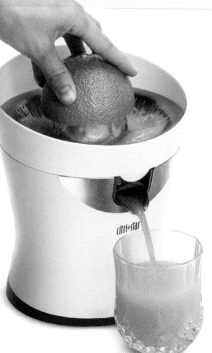

Of course, it's not easy to test different juicers before you buy one. As an alternative, you can watch an online video of me assembling and disassembling my favorite juicers. This will give you an idea of which juicer may be easiest for you to work with. Visit 7DayJustJuiceDiet.com.

Effort

Another consideration is how much physical force it takes to use your juicer. The triturators and masticating twin-gear machines require more pressure when inserting hard vegetables, such as carrots, than the high-speed centrifugal machines. Both types of machines, however, are labor intensive when it comes to juicing greens. But I'll give you some pointers on page 33 to make these processes easier.

Can't Buy a Juicer?

If you don't have a fruit and vegetable juicer and can't buy one now, you can still do this program. Here's how:

- If you're lucky enough to have a good juice bar nearby, you'll be able to purchase fresh-squeezed fruit and vegetable juice and wheatgrass juice. Some natural food stores have in-store juice bars, so check the ones near you.
- Buy frozen wheatgrass juice. The cubes melt easily in a glass with a little water and are still very potent. (See the information on frozen wheatgrass juice on page 23.)
- Drink the green juice from powder recommended on page 127, along with teas, vegetable broths, fresh apple cider, and homemade citrus juice.
- Invest in a good citrus juicer. Even the electric models are affordable, and they'll serve you well.

Size and Cost

A juicer's size and price might determine your final decision as much as anything. Even though you may crave an expensive machine, your budget might restrict you. If you have a tiny kitchen, you might be able to accommodate only a small juicer. And these priorities may conflict; for example, a vertically oriented slow juicer has a relatively small footprint, but is pricier than the bigger standard models.

Watch Sproutman demonstrate the assembly and disassembly of some of his favorite juicers.

HOW TO JUICE: TIPS AND TRICKS FOR SUCCESSFUL JUICING

Everybody wants the process of juicing to be fast and easy, but "easy juicing" is a health nut's oxymoron. It's actually a bit like saying "no-sweat snow shoveling." Both tasks are pretty basic, but they both require effort, and aren't you glad juicing is the less strenuous of the two! Now that you have that in perspective, here are some tips to make juicing easier.

Preparation

Perhaps the most time-consuming part of juicing is the prep and cleanup. Some veggies are prewashed; these will be the quickest to process. On the other hand, the veggies you just got fresh off the farm will need much more cleaning. I recommend filling the kitchen sink or a big bowl with water and giving these veggies a good soak and rinse.

Some people like to add disinfectants, such as hydrogen peroxide, white vinegar, or grapefruit seed extract, to the wash water (all of these products are available in most natural food stores). There are also commercial vege-

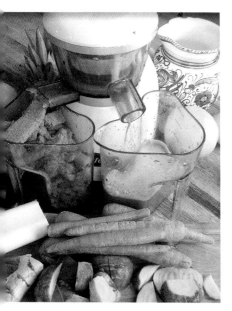

table wash products that claim to remove harmful bacteria and even waxes and pesticides. I just wash everything well in clean water and don't use any special products. But if you're more comfortable with the idea of using a disinfectant, you can find the most popular commercial brands among the resources listed on page 127.

Keep ease of preparation in mind when selecting veggies. You want the washing to be quick, not a whole separate side project. So, for example, buy carrots that are straight, thin, and clean instead of ones that are thick, gnarly, and dirty. Remember that the produce you juice doesn't need to be as blemish-free as produce you eat. Don't worry about cutting out blemishes and trimming tops and ends; the majority of them will ultimately get discarded in the pulp.

If any of your produce is too large to fit whole into your juicer's feed chute, cut it up into the largest pieces that will slide through the chute. It's fine to use stalks and stems that you might not normally eat because they're too tough. They still contain nutrients and will release some liquid.

Operation

As you gain more experience using your juicer, you'll learn how to feed in the fruits and vegetables to keep the process moving steadily. Anyone can clog any juicer by shoving in too much too fast. So take it slow. And keep in mind that some types of vegetables and fruits need special attention.

LEAFY VEGETABLES. Switch up the order when using green, leafy veggies, which are the hardest to juice. When you're feeding veggies through the shoot, alternate greens with stiff vegetables, such as carrots, celery, and beets. Try this sequence, for example: first put in some spinach, then a carrot, then more spinach, then a stalk of celery, then spinach again, and so on.

CARROTS. Wash carrots well before juicing, but don't obsess about scrubbing them perfectly clean, because the fiber is ejected by the machine. Match

Foam Happens

Don't foam with anger when you see foam in your juice! Some vegetables, such as beets, spinach, and kale, generate more foam than others during juicing. And some juicing machines are more prone to making foam.

It's difficult to drink foam, of course, but there's no harm in doing so. Simply stir as much foam as possible back into the juice to make it easier to consume. Or strain the juice. Some juicers come with strainers that help separate out the foam.

the size of your carrots to the size of the feed chute on your machine. You don't want to spend lots of time slicing carrots to fit them through the chute if you can avoid it.

BEETS. Be careful washing and juicing beets. The red splatter can make a mess, and no fabric in the world is immune to the dye of a red beet!

APPLES. Choose apples that juice easily and are likely to complement other ingredients. For example, Granny Smith apples are slightly preferred for juicing over other varieties because they are firm, tart, low in calories, and contain lots of antioxidants.

CITRUS FRUITS. All auger-style juicers can juice citrus fruits, but you'll need to peel, cut, and stuff the pieces down the juicing chute just as you would a carrot. Standard electric citrus juicers are faster and more convenient. But the single-auger juicers can juice the white pulpy part of the fruit, which contains a wealth of flavonoids.

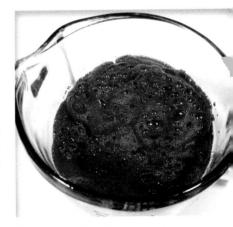

The foam on top of beet juice is as sweet as sugar.

Cleanup

Cleaning the juicer is something to take seriously. Don't put it aside for later or the task will only become more difficult. Quickly rinse all the machine parts; they should come clean easily. The only part of your juicer that should require more time and effort during cleaning is the screen; it takes a bit of patience to brush the tiny screen holes clean. If you no longer have the cleaning brush that came with your juicer, a new firm toothbrush will do the trick.

What About All That Pulp?

If you hate to waste anything, you might find it difficult to throw away all the pulp that's left over after juicing. After all, you spent good money on all those vegetables! But don't worry. You just extracted and consumed all the valuable nutrients that were in that produce. If you can, compost the pulp and contribute to the natural cycle of life by replenishing next season's garden.

If you're out of time and on the run, drop the screen into a bowl of water and let it soak. Brush it clean later. If you let the screen dry out, it will become encrusted with hard-to-remove juice fibers. Cleaning it at that point will be a tortuous task, and if any portions of the screen remain blocked, the flow of juice and the effectiveness of your juicer will be limited.

STORING AND TRANSPORTING FRESH JUICE

In an ideal world, you would drink fresh juice immediately after it's been made. But drinking fresh juice several times a day would then require multiple daily juicing sessions. For many folks, that's just not realistic. If you're going to succeed on this diet, you'll need to take advantage of efficiencies where you can, and that may involve minor trade-offs. After all, you don't want to make perfection the enemy of the good.

I find one of the best time-savers is to have a marathon juicing session, juicing one or two days' worth of drinks at once. You might hesitate to do this because the nutrients in juice are fragile and can easily degrade when exposed to air, warmth, and light. However, here are some tips that will protect your juice and enable you to juice less but drink more.

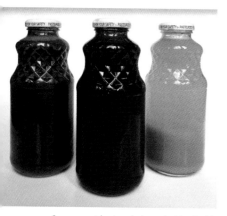

Green, carrot-beet, and pineapple juice freshly squeezed, filled to the very top, and chilled.

MINIMIZE EXPOSURE TO AIR. Get some 16-ounce (500-milliliter) glass bottles, preferably with tight lids. Make enough juice to fill several bottles to the very top. Leaving any air in the bottles will promote oxidation and the deterioration of nutrients. Cap off the bottles and put them in the freezer temporarily (see below). If you don't have enough juice to fill the last bottle up to the top, don't put it in the freezer; instead, drink the juice immediately or chill it in the refrigerator and drink it as soon as possible.

STRAIN OUT SEDIMENT. Not only will you digest your juice more quickly if it's been strained, but your juice will also keep longer because it's purer. So go ahead and strain it before bottling.

KEEP IT COLD. Don't be nervous when I say to put the bottled fresh juice in the freezer temporarily. You don't want to completely freeze the juice, as that would alter it and partially reduce its vitality. The freezer is only a temporary holding area to quickly reduce the temperature. You want to quickly chill the fresh juice, not freeze it solid. Aim for a temperature of about 36 degrees F (2 degrees C). You'll need a thermometer to know when the juice has dropped to the right temperature. Almost any kind of thermometer will do, but I recommend a digital infrared, point-and-shoot style thermometer. This type works quickly, is easy to use, and is available online and in some electronics stores.

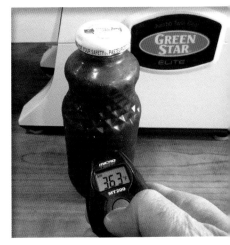

Fill your juice bottle to the very top and chill it to 36 degrees F (2 degrees C).

It may take 30 minutes or more for the juice to cool. (Using a timer will help you keep track of the time so you can avoid freezing your juice inadvertently.) Once it has cooled, transfer the bottles from the freezer to the refrigerator. If you want to drink your juice when you're away from home, pack it properly: chill an empty thermos and pour the cold juice into it. Store the thermos in the refrigerator until you're ready to walk out the door.

Oh, and one other thing. It's not a bad idea to check the refrigerator's temperature. Keeping it at the recommended range of 36 to 40 degrees F (2 degrees to 4.5 degrees C) will prolong the viability of your juices and fresh foods.

AVOID LIGHT. It's actually dark inside your refrigerator. Really! I know you might find this hard to believe because every time you look inside the refrigerator, there is light. But you just have to take a leap of faith that it really does go dark in there when you're not looking. This lack of light makes the refrigerator an ideal spot for storing juice.

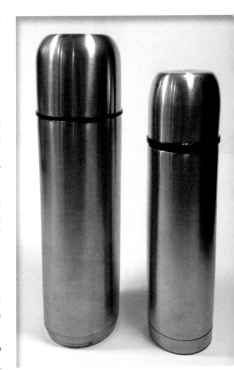

A high-quality thermos will keep your juice cold while you're on the go.

WATCH THE TIME. Even with all these precautions, you can only buy a limited amount of time before your juice degrades. How much time depends on how diligent you are in chilling your juice quickly and on the quality of your juicer. Slow juicers with built-in magnets and ceramics generate juice that will keep the longest: expect this juice to stay fresh for up to 48 hours after you make it. If you're getting close to the end of the 48-hour period and want to extend the viability of your juice for another day or so, put the juice bottles back in the freezer and chill them back down to 36 degrees F (2 degrees C), then immediately return the bottles to the fridge.

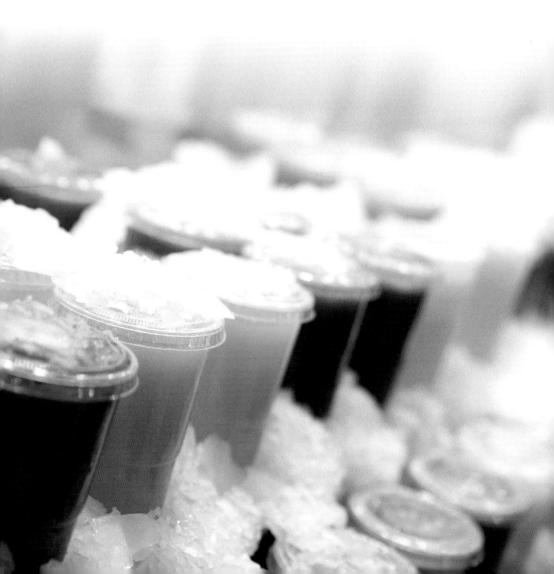

4

Planning Your Daily Routine

This chapter offers guidelines for how to structure your cleanse. I developed this framework, which includes a few options, based on feedback from the many people who have gone on my Just Juice Diet, as well as from my personal experience.

The juice diet can be modified to suit your needs. There's the Basic Plan, the Expanded Plan, and the Lite Plan. You'll find that within these plans there are a number of options. My diet program is extremely flexible; don't feel that you're unable to proceed because one particular step is too difficult for you.

START WITH A PRE-FAST DIET

One of the challenges many folks have when beginning a fast is getting over the hunger they feel during the first few days. You should find it easier to adjust to fasting if you transition gradually from your regular diet. I prepare my digestive system by eating light meals for one to three days leading up to the fast.

The best pre-fast diet is vegan, consisting of salads with simple dressings, fruits, vegetables, light soups, raw nuts and seeds, and nutritious drinks, such as herbal teas, vegetable broths, and juices—anything that doesn't come in a box or can. Sea vegetables, such as kelp, nori, and dulse, are also a great addition. Any of the post-fast recipes (pages 118 to 124), which will help you make the transition back to solid food after the fast, are also appropriate for the pre-fast diet.

What to Eat on Your Pre-Fast Diet

During the days preceding your Just Juice Diet, choose light and nourishing foods:

- raw fruits and vegetables
- fresh salads with simple dressings
- light vegan soups
- raw nuts and seeds
- teas, vegetable broths, and juices

If you're up for it, eliminate all cooking; keep everything you eat during this time fresh and raw. Not only does a raw vegan diet ease you into your week of just juice, but it also gives you a head start on the cleansing process.

Just as it's important to begin your fast gently, it's important to end it with a gradual transition back to solid foods. This is an extensive topic, so I've dedicated an entire chapter to it (see chapter 6).

A TYPICAL DAY

Here is the structure of the Basic Plan, but let's face it, each person is different and no matter what I recommend, everyone has individual needs and comfort levels. Our lives are not equally demanding, and we won't all be devoting ourselves equally to this effort. But this program is flexible enough to accommodate your particular situation.

- Drink 4 quarts (4 liters) total fluids during the day (see page 15).
- Add probiotic powder twice daily to fresh juice. I recommend a total of 50 billion units per day, so make that 25 billion units per drink.
- Take milk of magnesia before bedtime if necessary to keep things flowing.
- Do enough aerobic exercise, such as walking on a treadmill or light running, to achieve a sweat.
- Rest, meditate, or take a power nap when fatigued.
- Keep a fasting diary (see page 51).

THREE WAYS TO DO THIS PROGRAM

The Just Juice Diet features three different plans, and one of them is sure to fit your needs: the Basic Plan, the Expanded Plan for those who want to do more and maximize their benefits, and the Lite Plan for those who find even the Basic Plan to be a stretch.

Basic Plan

The Basic Plan contains all the primary elements, essential drinks, and exercises you'll be doing on this program. This is the plan most people do.

Expanded Plan

The Expanded Plan is the same as the Basic Plan but includes additional cleansing activities, such as bathing, bodywork, and colonics. Maybe you'll begin and end your fast with a colonic (see page 65). You could also schedule some bodywork once or twice during the fast. Taking saunas or steam baths regularly is helpful, as is a daily hot bath featuring Epsom salts or powdered mustard (see resources, page 126).

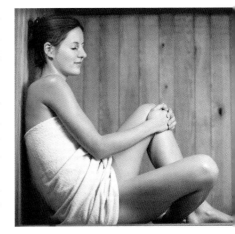

These additional therapies require more of your time and effort, but they can truly further the degree of detox you'll achieve and maximize the progress you'll make in one short week. You're a candidate for these extras if you have the time and energy, have access to some of these therapies, have had some prior experience with cleansing, and feel up to the challenge.

TABLE 2. Basic Plan

DRINKS	AMOUNT
Pure water (Water Flush)	1 quart (1 liter) daily
Fresh green vegetable juices	1 quart (1 liter) daily
Colon cleansers	1 quart (1 liter) daily
Other drinks	1 quart (1 liter), including 8 to 16 ounces (250 to 500 milliliters) of liver cleansers daily and no more than 16 ounces (500 milliliters) of sweet juice daily
Milk of magnesia	1 to 4 tablespoons (15 to 60 milliliters), as needed
Probiotics	50 billion units daily, divided into two doses, ideally added to fresh juice
Aerobic exercise	30 minutes daily

TABLE 3. Expanded Plan

DRINKS	AMOUNT
Pure water (Water Flush)	1 quart (1 liter) daily
Fresh green vegetable juices	1 quart (1 liter) daily
Colon cleansers	1 quart (1 liter) daily
Other drinks	1 quart (1 liter), including 8 to 16 ounces (250 to 500 milliliters) of liver cleansers daily and no more than 16 ounces (500 milliliters) of sweet juice daily
Milk of magnesia	1 to 4 tablespoons (15 to 60 milliliters), as needed
Probiotics	50 billion units daily, divided into two doses, ideally added to fresh juice
Aerobic exercise	30 minutes daily
Bodywork, such as massage, reflexology, or rolfing	See page 62.
Colonic	See page 63.
Footbath	See page 59.
Hot bath with Epsom salts or powdered mustard	See page 57.
Sauna or steam bath	See page 57.

Lite Plan

The Lite Plan is similar to the Basic Plan except it doesn't require juicing at home. It's the plan for you if you don't have a juicer or don't have time to juice. You can get fresh green vegetable juice from a local juice bar or mix green juices using high-quality green juice powder (see page 127). This plan is less nutritionally potent than the Basic or Extended Plans, but the workload is less taxing. Of course, you can also visit a juice bar and use green juice powder if you choose the Basic Plan. The Lite Plan simply provides more flexibility and a less intense regimen if you need it.

TABLE 4. Lite Plan

DRINKS	AMOUNT
Pure water (Water Flush)	1 quart (1 liter) daily
Fresh vegetable juice or juice mixed from green juice powder	1 quart (1 liter) daily
Colon cleansers	1 quart (1 liter) daily
Other drinks	1 quart (1 liter), including 8 ounces (250 milliliters) of liver cleansers daily and no more than 16 ounces (500 milliliters) of sweet juice daily
Probiotics	25 to 50 billion units daily, divided into two doses, ideally added to fresh juice
Aerobic exercise	20 to 30 minutes every other day

CREATE YOUR CLEANSING SCHEDULE

Many people have asked me over the years how I structure my day when I'm fasting. I find having a game plan is quite useful because it helps me remember to incorporate everything I want to do during the day. To this end, Sproutman's Daily Just Juice Diary (see page 52) is very helpful.

There are also advantages to doing certain things early in the day or late in the day. Table 5 (page 44) and table 6 (page 44), which represent a less ambitious and a more ambitious daily regimen, reflect this order. These tables are intended to be helpful examples, but you get to decide how you want to structure your day and fit everything in. For more suggestions, see "Divide the Day into Five Parts," page 45.

These timelines are just guides, and I expect you to customize them. You're the final judge as to what you're going to drink and when you're going to drink it. Are you in the mood for something sweet? Acidic? Green? Spicy? Follow your instincts. Your senses will actually become a little sharper during the fast, because you're not inundated with the usual volume of food, so examine how you feel. If your energy is low, choose one of the sweet juices; they add quick energy. If you're feeling actual fatigue, don't stimulate yourself with sugar. Rest instead. Take a meditation break or a power nap to recharge your batteries. After you rest, maybe have a green vegetable juice. Green juices produce long-term energy because they're powerfully nourishing.

TABLE 5. A less ambitious day, drinking 3 quarts (3 liters) of liquid

8:00 a.m.	Water Flush: Drink pure water, 1 quart (1 liter), in 20 minutes
9:00 a.m.	Drink Grapefruit Liver Cleanser (page 111), 8 ounces (250 milliliters)
10:00 a.m.	Exercise for 30 minutes
11:00 a.m.	Drink green vegetable juice with probiotics, ½ quart (500 milliliters)
2:00 p.m.	Drink colon cleanser, ½ quart (500 milliliters)
4:00 p.m.	Drink your choice from Other Drinks (see page 20), ½ quart (500 milliliters)
7:00 p.m.	Drink green vegetable juice with probiotics, ½ quart (500 milliliters)
10:00 p.m.	Drink herbal tea, 8 ounces (250 milliliters)
11:00 p.m.	Take milk of magnesia, 1 to 4 tablespoons (15 to 60 milliliters)

You'll need to consume fiber to keep things moving, and on the Just Juice Diet, colon cleansers will be your primary source of fiber. I recommend two 16-ounce (500-milliliter) colon-cleansing drinks per day, one in the morning and another in the afternoon (see sidebar, page 45). You can prepare 1 quart (1 liter) at once to save time; store the two portions in two separate bottles.

TABLE 6. A more ambitious day, drinking 4½ quarts (4½ liters) of liquid

8:00 a.m.	Water Flush: Drink pure water, 1 quart (1 liter), in 20 minutes
9:00 a.m.	Drink Grapefruit Liver Cleanser (page 111), ½ quart (500 milliliters)
10:00 a.m.	Drink colon cleanser, ½ quart (500 milliliters)
11:00 a.m.	Exercise for 30 minutes
12:00 noon	Drink green vegetable juice with probiotics, ½ quart (500 milliliters)
2:00 p.m.	Drink your choice from Other Drinks (see page 20), ½ quart (500 milliliters)
4:00 p.m.	Drink colon cleanser, ½ quart (500 milliliters)
5:00 p.m.	Meditate
6:00 p.m.	Drink green vegetable juice with probiotics, ½ quart (500 milliliters)
8:00 p.m.	Drink hot vegetable broth, 8 ounces (250 milliliters)
10:00 p.m.	Drink herbal tea, 8 ounces (250 milliliters)
10:30 p.m.	Take a hot Epsom salt bath
11:00 p.m.	Take milk of magnesia, 1 to 4 tablespoons (15 to 60 milliliters)

About Colon-Cleansing Drinks

Colon cleansers have certain characteristics that you should consider when planning your daily schedule during the Just Juice Diet.

- A colon-cleansing drink (see recipes pages 107 to 110) forms a mucilage that traps most nutrients. For this reason, it's a good idea to wait one hour after drinking a colon cleanser before consuming fresh vegetable juice.

- A colon-cleansing drink made from flaxseeds or psyllium seeds is viscous, so it's always beneficial to follow it with a glass of water.

- If you plan to be out and about, colon-cleansing drinks are very portable. Because they're not as perishable as fresh juice, they don't need to be kept cool in a thermos.

Sometimes I prepare two days' worth of colon-cleansing drinks at once because unlike juice, these drinks are not perishable.

Every day during the fast you may feel different. Some days you might have less ambition and won't feel up to the task of drinking something every hour or two. If you're not able to drink the entire 4 quarts (4 liters) of liquids I suggest, don't beat yourself up! Just do the best you can. You have the freedom to relax your schedule, as in the less ambitious day (see table 5, page 44). At the same time, it's important to know when to push yourself. After all, you're doing this to get results. If you take on the more ambitious schedule (see table 6, page 44), you'll make more progress.

DIVIDE THE DAY INTO FIVE PARTS

When structuring your time during the 7-Day Just Juice Diet, it might be helpful to think of the day as having five parts: morning, afternoon, evening, bedtime, and any time in between. Reserve different parts of the day for certain drinks or activities. Remember, though, that the following sections, like table 5 (page 44) and table 6 (page 44), provide suggestions. While the Water Flush is certainly best to do first thing, ultimately you decide when you want to drink most drinks, when you want to exercise, and when you want to fit in optional therapies.

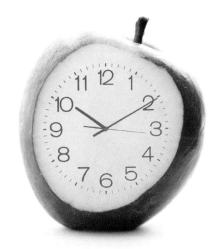

Morning

Mornings are often busy, and you may be wondering how you're going to have time for the juice fast, especially if you have to leave for work. Preparing your drinks in advance is the best solution. It's also possible that you may not get to do everything on the list every morning. But the more you can do, the more effective your cleanse will be.

Cleansing begins shortly after rising with the Water Flush, which means drinking down 1 quart (1 liter) of water within 20 minutes. That volume of liquid exceeds the capacity of the urinary tract, and the excess is rerouted through the intestinal tract, so the water flushes both systems. Think of it as a colonic from the top down.

What if you have no morning bowel movement? Bring out the milk of magnesia. As shown in table 5 (page 44) and table 6 (page 44), I recommend a dose at bedtime. However, if the morning comes without any benefit, you could take a repeat dose in the morning. Flow is what a cleanse is all about, and the sole purpose of this product is to promote that flow, so add it to your morning routine if your intestines aren't cooperating. Remember: movement promotes health; congestion promotes disease.

Movement promotes health; congestion promotes disease.

About an hour after finishing the Water Flush, I drink a Grapefruit Liver Cleanser (page 111)—one of my favorites. It's easy to make, delicious, and mild but effective. Sure, there are other liver detox drinks, and even entire programs, that are more intense. Some programs take a whole week and are capable of eliminating both liver stones and gallstones. The Grapefruit Liver

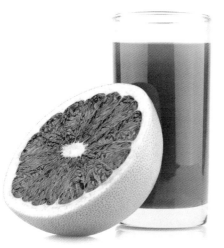

Cleanser, however, is designed to provide a mild and gradual cleanse, which is why you'll want to drink it daily. To maximize the cleanser's effectiveness, wait at least one hour after drinking it before drinking anything else. Although it's not mandatory to drink the Grapefruit Liver Cleanser in the morning, I recommend it. Cleansing your liver is a great way to start off the day. I also recommend drinking a colon cleanser in the morning. During the next hour, I drink a carrot-beet juice—one that I made in advance and stored—if I'm in the mood for something sweet. On a less ambitious day, however, I might just have a green vegetable juice late in the morning.

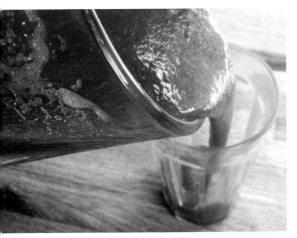

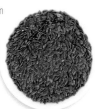

Colon-cleansing drinks made from either psyllium seeds or flaxseeds can get quite viscous, as visible in this psyllium, water, and prune juice mixture. That's why you should blend it and wait 5 to 8 minutes before drinking it. Letting it thicken in the blender is better than having it thicken in your stomach. Add extra water to thin it so it's easy to drink, and use prune juice, coconut water, or your favorite juice to make it pleasing to your palate.

I suggest the following steps to help you meet your goals and organize your time early in the day:

- Do the Water Flush by drinking 1 quart (1 liter) of pure, room-temperature water. Drink it all down in 20 minutes.
- Take milk of magnesia (1 to 4 tablespoons or 15 to 60 milliliters), if needed.
- Drink a Grapefruit Liver Cleanser (page 111) (8 to 16 ounces or 250 to 500 milliliters).
- Drink a colon cleanser (16 ounces or 500 milliliters).
- And if you have the time and appetite, drink fresh-squeezed sweet juice made from pineapple, carrots, apples, beets, grapes, or watermelon. Mix your probiotics into this juice.

Ask Sproutman

Dear Sproutman: You mention making the colon cleanser with flaxseeds or psyllium seeds. Could I also prepare it with chia seeds? —*Selina*

Dear Selina: True, chia seeds, like psyllium seeds and flaxseeds, become gelatinous in liquid, providing the needed consistency for a colon cleanser. So the short answer is yes. And what's more, chia seeds also taste good! So why don't I recommend them? Putting on my pragmatist hat, I must note that chia seeds are three to four times more pricey than the other two seeds. In addition, chia seeds create only about half as much viscosity as flaxseeds when added to liquid. So, more money, less gel are the reasons I'm underwhelmed about using chia seeds for this purpose.

Afternoon

You need to drink 1 quart (1 liter) of fresh green vegetable juice daily. I suggest splitting this into two 16-ounce (500-milliliter) portions and consuming one in the afternoon and one in the evening. But you can drink green vegetable juice anytime that suits you, and you can also drink more than I recommend. Again, green vegetable juice is the most nutritious and healing drink in this program, so enjoy as much of it as possible.

If you're out and about and don't happen to have a thermos full of fresh green vegetable juice with you, green juice powder is your alternative. Although green juice made from powder isn't as nutritious, it offers portability and and convenience, and there are some high-quality brands available. (For recommendations, see resources, page 127.)

Afternoon might be a good time of day for you to make up a batch of fresh green vegetable juice. You can make more juice than you need and store the leftovers for later by following my storing and chilling suggestions on page 36.

You can exercise anytime that best suits your schedule, but do it. Exercise is a key part of this program; you cannot accomplish the cleanse with drinks alone. For more information about exercise, see page 56.

Include the following on your list of afternoon goals:

- Drink fresh green vegetable juice (16 ounces or 500 milliliters).
- Drink a colon cleanser, followed by a glass of water.
- Exercise.

Evening

Your evening routine could simply include drinking a green vegetable juice, colon cleanser, and some hot tea. Here's your list:

- Drink green vegetable juice (16 ounces or 500 milliliters). Mix probiotics into the juice.
- Drink a colon cleanser (16 ounces or 500 milliliters).
- Drink hot tea, vegetable broth, or another hot drink.

Bedtime

Late in the evening, just before bed, is the ideal time to take a hot bath. Learn about the benefits of a hot bath with Epsom salts or powdered mustard and how to prepare one on page 57. This is the week to give yourself a little extra time, attention, and care, and relaxing in a hot bath is one way of doing just that. Your body works hard for you all year; give it the love and attention it deserves! Bedtime is also the ideal time to drink plenty of water and take a dose of milk of magnesia. Here's your bedtime list:

- Take a hot bath. Make it extra cleansing by adding Epsom salts or powdered mustard.
- Drink pure water in any amount that you want.
- Take milk of magnesia, as needed.

Any Time

While certain drinks should be taken at specific times, others are perfect any time of the day. For example, you can grab something from the "Optional Drinks" list (page 22), such as coconut water, kombucha, or aloe vera juice.

In addition, mix up a drink with green juice powder whenever you want. Green juice powder is an essential part of my Lite Plan for those who need the convenience. Because drinks made from green juice powder are portable and nonperishable, they're great when you're on the run. Here's your list:

- Choose any of the optional drinks I recommend.
- Mix up a drink using green juice powder whenever you need something convenient.

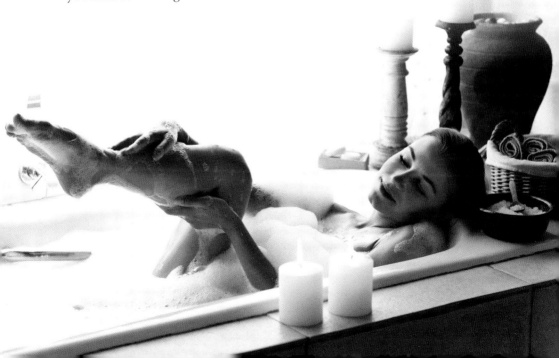

When to Use Probiotics

I recommend using probiotic powder (see resources, page 126), which can be mixed into drinks, preferably fresh juices. However, it's okay to use probiotic capsules during the pre-fast diet. It's best to take two doses of probiotics each day, such as in the morning and the evening. For the best results, mix probiotic powder with sweet juice. It's good to take probiotics with sweet juices because the bacteria will feed on the sugar. In addition, probiotics can also be added to fresh green vegetable juice.

Whatever you do, don't take probiotics with hot drinks; heat will destroy the beneficial organisms. Also, I don't recommend adding probiotics to colon-cleansing drinks, because the bacteria are likely to get trapped by the mucilage in the drink and ride their way out of your digestive tract without ever benefiting you. Considering that probiotics are expensive, I like to play it safe and keep all live nutrients and friendly bacteria away from the psyllium and flaxseed drinks.

Ask Sproutman

Dear Sproutman: I was unable to find a probiotic powder. Can I empty out the powder from capsules into my drinks or is it okay to take the capsules? —*Janice*

Dear Janice: Capsules are not my first choice, but they're acceptable temporarily. Sure, you can open them up and pour out the probiotic powder, even though that's a hassle. The capsule itself is not a lot to digest, but you'll be gulping down many of them during the day and they add up. Also, some capsules are designed to resist digestion so the probiotics will travel deeper into your intestines. If necessary, use capsules to start, but get powdered probiotics as soon as possible.

When to Take Milk of Magnesia

Start taking milk of magnesia gradually if you need a laxative to encourage a bowel movement. Begin with 1 tablespoon (15 milliliters) per night and increase the dose by 1 tablespoon each night until you get a response. You can use up to 4 tablespoons (60 milliliters) at night if that's how much it takes to promote a bowel movement the next morning. You can take 1 additional tablespoon in the morning if nothing is moving. Increase the dose gradually, however; milk of magnesia can cause diarrhea if you use too much. Also, it's okay to take a break from it. Tune into your body and decide if you need a day off. You may find that you're getting good intestinal flow without it.

SCHEDULE TIME TO REST AND RECORD

You may be thinking that you already have enough to do during the 7-Day Just Juice Diet. I hear you! But if you can manage it, I highly recommend reserving time for not just a full night's sleep but also plenty of additional rest. Also helpful is jotting down your impressions as they come to you.

Sleep and Rest

A good amount of healing takes place when you sleep. Manage your sleep well this week because the more rest you get, the more reserves you'll have for inner cleaning. Many people report that they need less sleep during the Just Juice Diet, and this is indeed one of the benefits of fasting. Since you're not expending energy on digestion, you may feel too energized to sleep! If that's the case, a hot Epsom salt bath before bedtime may be just the thing to help you nod off.

It's also important to rest when you feel fatigued instead of reaching for some caffeine. Take a power nap or a meditation break to reduce fatigue and stress. Remember that stress is a contributing factor to nearly every major disease.

Keep a Diary

I mentioned earlier that you may hit a few difficult moments during the cleanse. You might also find it difficult to keep track of what and how much you've had to drink and what cleansing activities you've done throughout the week. One way to track your challenges and remember what you've done is to keep a diary.

I've provided a template (page 52) that you can copy to create a diary, or you can print a similar form from 7DayJustJuiceDiet.com or scan the QR code on this page. Since this is a daily diary, copy or print one sheet for each day. The daily diary makes it easy to monitor yourself. You can look back and see how you're doing and improve any areas of insufficiency. Also, you can record whether you're having discomfort or feeling great. Your diary entries document the

Just Juice diary template.

whole process you're going through, especially your emotions. This written record can help you and anyone you're consulting with diagnose what's going on and make any necessary corrections.

Sproutman's Daily Just Juice Diary

DAY 1 2 3 4 5 6 7 (CIRCLE ONE)		TODAY'S DATE:		
DAILY FLUIDS				
	8 OZ / 250 ML	16 OZ / 500 ML	1 QUART / 1 LITER	TOTAL
Green vegetable juice				
Grapefruit Liver Cleanser				
Colon cleanser				
Sweet juice				
Water				
Other drinks				

EXTRAS				
Probiotics	a.m.	p.m.		billions
Milk of magnesia	# of tablespoons			

EXERCISE

MEASUREMENTS

Sleep (# of hours)	Sleep quality
Comments:	
Bowel movements (#)	Time(s) of day
Comments:	

OTHER ACTIVITIES

Massage

Sauna

Colonic

OPTIONAL MEASUREMENTS

Blood pressure	Fasting blood sugar level

5

Optimizing Your Detoxification

Detoxification is hard work. A lot of this work is conducted in your intestines. After all, your intestines zigzag like a roller coaster and would stretch out to a full thirty feet if they were untangled. If something gets stuck in this long and winding tract, you can't see it or reach it. You can only flush it out. That's why we use colon cleansers, colonics, and vegetable juices that act like solvents to detox the digestive tract.

The body, however, is more than just plumbing. You've also got major organs, not to mention fatty tissues, glands, and trillions of cells, to clean. How are you going to reach them? The answer is simple: focus on general detoxification activities that will have a system-wide effect. Some therapies help to detox lots of parts, and that information is front and center in this chapter. Use it to prevent the recirculation of the scuzz that causes headaches and saps your energy.

On the other hand, you can take some targeted actions to pamper certain organs. We have five primary organs and systems that need detoxification: the lungs, liver, skin, intestines, and urinary tract (kidneys and bladder). I call these organs my closest friends. I want to take good care of them, just as I care for my family, because their welfare is my lifeline. I'll do some cleansing for each of these beloved organs. I'll flush and massage them and squeeze and scour them. It's spring-cleaning time.

Let's think about what that means for a moment. When cleaning your house, you vacuum and mop the floors and dust the bookshelves and wall hangings. You loosen up a lot of dirt. You might start coughing and sneezing and your eyes may start to water—these are the consequences of a good cleaning. Once you begin unleashing the cobwebs and crud—either in your house or your body—you inevitably release a maelstrom of muck and mire!

Not to worry. When you clean your house, you turn on the exhaust fan and open the doors and windows to clear away the fallout. And that's essentially what you do with your body during a cleansing fast. I'm going to teach you how to use a number of different techniques and practices that will maximize your efforts to flush out and release harmful toxins. Your mission is to release and eject. First you detox, then you discharge.

OVERALL DETOXIFICATION

Although juices are at the core of my detox program, there's a limit to how much you can accomplish by drinking juice. For the best results, you must also use several other tools, techniques, and practices to maximize detoxification. Some of these, including exercise, hot baths, footbaths, and saunas, influence multiple organs or have a system-wide effect.

AEROBIC EXERCISE FOR OVERALL DETOXING

Exercise benefits all five organs of detoxification. That's why it's a required daily practice during the 7-Day Just Juice Diet. Your focus should be on aerobic exercise, such as biking, walking, dancing, jogging, and swimming. Tai chi and yoga are not considered aerobic, but these activities achieve similar results by manipulating, pressing, and squeezing the muscles and tissues to release toxins. Jumping on a trampoline, also known as rebounding, is ideal for stimulating lymphatic circulation.

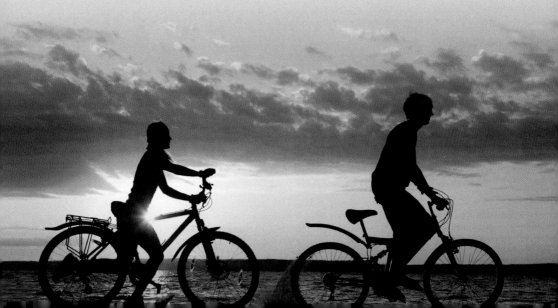

LOVE YOUR LYMPH

T he key to detoxification is your lymphatic system. While the circulatory system with its big heart typically gets all the attention, your lymphatic system is quietly doing all the hard work of keeping you clean. What is the lymphatic system? It's a network of vessels that transports the waste products of cellular metabolism, including white blood cells and lymphocytes that fight bacteria, viruses, and even cancer. While you're on the Just Juice Diet and drinking lots of water and phytochemical-rich, highly solvent juices, you release toxins from your tissues, organs, and glands at an increased rate. During this time, it's essential that you make your lymphatic system as efficient as possible. Otherwise, you'll just end up recirculating toxins instead of releasing them.

Unlike the circulatory system with its pumping heart, the lymphatic system must rely on the contractions of your muscles or pressure from external forces in order to circulate. Exercise such as yoga or jumping on a trampoline— anything that squeezes, massages, manipulates, or moves your body—will stimulate and improve the health of your lymphatic system.

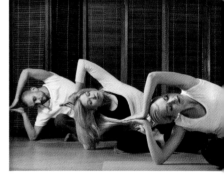

As a general rule during the juice fast, choose gentle activities, such as yoga, that invigorate, stimulate, and circulate, rather than activities that burn and enervate. Manage your energy so your organs and glands can do their inner housekeeping.

So, what if you're accustomed to more strenuous exercise? If you're a regular runner, you can continue to run during the juice cleanse—just don't run like you're training for a marathon. If you're a weight lifter, this is not the week to build muscles. When you develop muscle, you need to push your body hard and eat protein. Save bodybuilding for another time. This is a week of detoxification, so you should be in a catabolic (breaking-down) cycle rather than an anabolic (building-up) cycle. Muscle building is actually counterproductive during detox, because your body is busy breaking down fatty tissue and squeezing out poisons. This should be a week of "innercise," rather than extreme exercise.

This should be a week of "innercise," rather than extreme exercise.

Cleansing Your Lungs and Skin

Exercising is particularly beneficial for the lungs and skin. You normally breathe about fourteen to eighteen times per minute, but during exercise

Exercise Every Day

It's essential to keep moving during the juice fast to release toxins. These are some helpful activities:

- biking
- jumping on a trampoline
- low-impact dancing or movement
- light jogging/running

- swimming
- tai chi
- walking (outdoors or on a treadmill)
- yoga

that range may easily be doubled, as your lungs work harder and expel a greater volume of gases. Your lungs are critical to your detox because they're the fastest route to your bloodstream. The air sacs in your lungs are lined with capillary beds that feed directly into the pulmonary vein. Increased breathing from exercise bathes your cells in oxygen, and your exhalations simultaneously exhaust greater amounts of gases. When you exercise, you efficiently expel the waste products of cellular metabolism.

Perspiration is an amazing process. Your skin is made up of two to four million sweat glands, and you can potentially sweat out as much as 2 quarts (2 liters) of waste-filled fluid in an hour! Exercise heats up your

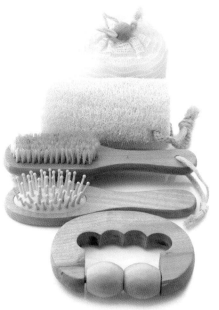

muscles and causes them to excrete more waste products in the form of water, salt, lactic acid, and urea. These all exit through the sweat glands, which can result in a distinctly unpleasant odor. This is your body's natural cleaning mechanism, so the week of your juice fast is a good time to ratchet up the sweat.

Exercise that induces perspiration helps alleviate skin rashes and conditions, such as eczema, because it promotes more cleansing through the skin's layers. Quite simply, if you sweat more on a regular basis, you'll have healthier skin. When not exercising, you can still stimulate your pores by gently brushing your skin. This opens the pores and increases circulation. You can use either a skin brush or a loofah sea sponge; both can be found in large natural food stores. Wearing breathable clothes is also important, as many synthetic fabrics are actually derived from plastics that can inhibit dermal respiration.

Therapies for Skin Cleansing

Don't forget that your skin is your largest organ, and it requires extra care during your cleanse. Suggested activities include the following:

- exercise
- massage
- sauna or steam bath
- skin brushing
- skin exposure to sunlight (without sunburn)

OTHER TREATMENTS FOR OVERALL DETOXIFICATION

There's a lot you can do to detox beyond drinking juice and exercising. Table 3, page 42, outlines what I call the "expanded" version of the 7-Day Just Juice Diet. This part of the program is considered optional, but it involves cleansing activities that are very beneficial. If you have the time or inclination, this is the week to get a massage, sit in a sauna, or take advantage of the services at your local health spa. There are a number of things you can try, but because sweating is so detoxifying, any treatment that increases perspiration should be on your list. I like to have a daily sauna, for example, but if that's not possible for you, get an ionic footbath or simply take a hot bath in your own tub—just add Epsom salts or powdered mustard.

When muscles and tissues are manipulated and squeezed, blood and lymph circulate more and offload more waste products. For example, if a bodyworker is mechanically massaging your intestines, you can be sure things will start to move! When skin pores are heated by a sauna, far infrared sauna, or steam bath, they open and release lymphatic fluid to help you achieve a deeper cleanse. All these treatments increase your rate of detoxification.

Hot Baths

People have been using mineral baths for hydrotherapy since ancient times. More recently, former US president Franklin Delano Roosevelt regularly used hydrotherapy to relieve the effects of polio. You can find health spas and sanatoriums all over the world in places where hot, mineral-rich water emerges from deep below the surface of the earth to create spring-fed pools, providing opportunities for people to heal and recuperate.

So what is the secret? Why is hydrotherapy so effective? The answer lies in the saltiness of the water. When you're in salty water, the less salty fluids in your body are naturally pulled toward the saltier water, whether it's

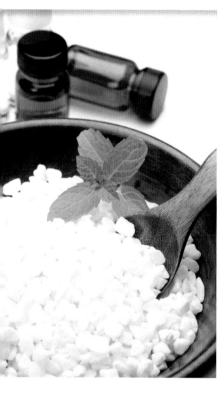

in the pool, bathtub, a natural spring, or even the sea. The Dead Sea is one very famous example of a body of salty water that people soak in to treat asthma, psoriasis, osteoporosis, and more. (It's so salty, bathers float rather than sink!)

An Epsom salt bath is one of my favorite treatments, because the salt is affordable and very effective, and most people have access to a bathtub. Epsom salts mimic the effect of a natural hot spring. Composed of magnesium sulfite, the salts are naturally derived from the mineral epsomite. The magnesium in the Epsom salts can soothe and relax muscles and will do wonders for relieving stress and even lowering blood pressure. Epsom salts can also be taken internally as a purgative to flush the intestines.

Simply sitting in a hot tub that's about 10 degrees F (5.5 degrees C) hotter than your body temporarily elevates your temperature to the level it would be if you were running a fever. Since a fever is the body's natural mechanism for expelling bacteria and viruses, mimicking a fever is perfect for a cleanse. This process of temperature elevation is called hyperthermia and is even used as a cancer therapy.

Another effective bath ingredient is powdered mustard, and I recommend a product called Dr. Singha's Mustard Bath (see resources, page 126). The mustard bath is an age-old remedy that heats up the skin and opens the pores. Mustard is very stimulating, cleansing, and rejuvenating. When you sit in a mustard bath, you'll feel the heat generated by the mustard, and you'll have no doubt that you're sweating out lots of impurities. Like Epsom salts, powdered mustard is a great muscle relaxant; is excellent for skin conditions, tension, and joint soreness; and is a wonderful remedy for sleeplessness. Use

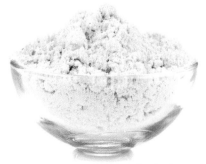

2 ounces (60 milliliters) of powdered mustard per bath and follow the directions for making a hyperthermia bath (see sidebar, page 59), replacing the Epsom salts with powdered mustard.

To take a hyperthermia bath, pour 2 to 3 pounds of Epsom salts into the tub and fill the tub halfway with tolerably hot water. Lie down in the tub and slowly continue to fill it with the hottest water you can stand, but no hotter than 110 degrees F (44 degrees C). Move the salt around until it dis-

Powdered mustard

Make a Hyperthermia Bath

1. Pour 2 to 3 pounds of Epsom salts into a bathtub.
2. Fill up the tub halfway with tolerably hot water.
3. Lie down in the tub.
4. Continue running the hot water slowly.
5. Make the water as hot as tolerable, with a maximum temperature of 110 degrees F (44 degrees C).
6. Optional: Place a cold cloth on your head or forehead.
7. Try to stay in the water for 20 minutes.
8. Optional: Rinse off in the shower.
9. Jump into bed under a warm blanket.

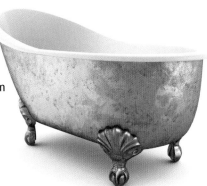

solves. Remain in the bath for at least 20 minutes. You can place a cold cloth over your head or forehead to help you stay comfortable. When you're done, rinse off briefly in the shower and dry off. Then jump right into bed under a warm blanket and rest for another 20 minutes. You'll still be sweating for most of that time as your body temperature slowly returns to normal.

The hyperthermia bath is a simple procedure that is greatly relaxing and very therapeutic. You can do it as frequently as once daily if you desire. It's especially useful when you're experiencing headaches and fatigue, and it even helps a fever by enhancing detoxification.

Footbaths

The soles of your feet are unique in that all your body's acupuncture meridians (energy pathways) converge there. This area is so important to good health and healing that there's a specific type of bodywork (called reflexology) devoted entirely to manipulating the feet and stimulating these meridians.

These energy pathways act as conduits for the lymphatic system. Because footbaths encourage the transfer of toxins through your skin into hot water that contains salt or powdered mustard, they're very

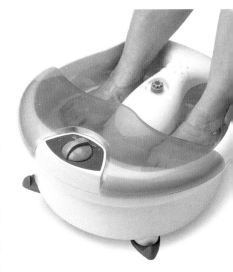

The ionic footbath uses a mild electric current to stimulate a detox through the feet.

Optional Therapies that Enhance Detoxification

The Enhanced Plan (see table 3, page 42), includes the following therapies:

- aerobic exercise
- bodywork (massage, reflexology, rolfing, etc.)
- colon hydrotherapy
- footbaths
- hot baths (with Epsom salts or powdered mustard)
- sauna (steam or far infrared)
- spa treatment

effective for enhancing detoxification. One type of footbath features a low-level electric current that runs through the water, although the current is too low for you to feel. This type of bath is called an ionic footbath because the current generates a magnetic pull that draws toxins out through the energy pathways in the feet, causing discoloration of the bathwater. Although the water turns somewhat brown because of the chemical reaction between the salt and the electricity, dark brown and green spots are also visible, and these are said to be pollutants from the liver and gallbladder. To test a footbath's effectiveness, dip a pH strip (the kind used to test urine) into the water before and after you use it. After your footbath, the pH should be more alkaline, which is the desired result.

THE LIVER

The liver is an amazing organ with hundreds of functions relating to metabolism, synthesizing nutrients, breaking down fats, regulating cholesterol, storing glucose and vitamins, and much more. It's arguably the most important organ for detoxification, and that's why you'll do liver cleansing daily on the Just Juice Diet. The liver is responsible for a long list of biochemical processes, such as detoxification, emulsification of fats, protein synthesis, and the breakdown of complex molecules from both food and pollutants. Improving the functionality of your liver could eliminate numerous insidious health problems, such as hepatitis, cirrhosis, jaundice, skin conditions, cancer, and gallstones, and add years to your life. No one has a perfectly functioning liver, but you can improve the functioning of yours by helping it expel its toxic load.

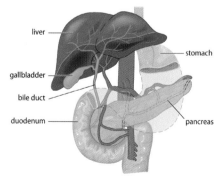

liver

gallbladder

bile duct

duodenum

stomach

pancreas

Detox Your Liver with . . .

- Apple Cider Vinegar Drink (page 112)
- Grapefruit Liver Cleanser (page 111)
- herbal teas
- Hot Lemon Tea (page 113)
- wheatgrass juice
- garlic or ginger added to vegetable juice
- a hot compress
- a liver massage
- yoga

Drinks

Lemon juice is a potent substance for liver health because of the cleansing effect of its main compound, limonene. My Grapefruit Liver Cleanser (page 111) contains lemon juice and is gentle, delicious, and effective. The liver also responds to heat, so Hot Lemon Tea (page 113) is very healing. Be sure to try the Apple Cider Vinegar Drink (page 112) to help the liver break down fats and promote the movement of bile.

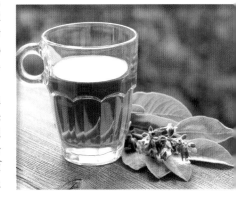

There are also a number of herbs that wield a powerful healing effect on the liver. Garlic helps the liver detoxify carcinogens before they can be spread to other parts of the body. It also can prevent fatty liver, lower cholesterol, and retard the formation of gallstones. Add garlic to any vegetable juice, lemon juice drink, or tea.

Ginger is another highly effective liver cleanser. Gingerol, the pungent compound in ginger, promotes the flow of bile, a necessary part of any cleanse. Ginger can also protect the liver against the toxic effects of alcohol and inhibit the development of liver cancer. Add ginger to your juices or make Hot Ginger Tea (page 114).

In addition, you can add hot herbal teas to your liver-cleansing arsenal. Herbs such as burdock, dandelion, milk thistle, and ginseng, as well as green tea, all stimulate bile secretion, reduce cholesterol, prevent gallstones, and protect against liver cancer. Teas that feature these individual herbs or a mixture are available wherever herbal remedies are sold.

Teas for the Liver

Hot teas stimulate the liver, and the following varieties are especially helpful:

- burdock
- dandelion
- ginseng
- green
- lemon
- licorice
- milk thistle
- schizandra
- turmeric

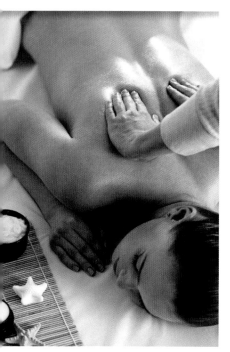

Exercise and Massage

Jumping on a trampoline is great exercise for the liver because it moves all your organs and frees them from the endless pull of gravity. Inversion exercises (such as headstands and shoulder stands in yoga), hanging upside down, and the use of inclined benches are also helpful.

Massage provides direct manipulation of the liver, increasing the circulation of blood and the release of waste products. Even using a handheld massage wand over the liver is helpful when you can't visit a bodyworker. An aggressive massage can be so effective that special care must be taken afterward to ensure that newly released toxins don't reenter the bloodstream. Scheduling a colonic after a vigorous liver massage would be ideal.

Hot Compresses

The use of a hot compress (the application of oil and heat) is a traditional remedy dating back to ancient Egypt. Even though they have fallen out of style, hot compresses are still effective. They can increase circulation, reduce inflammation, and promote detoxification. Although a hot compress is ideal for healing the liver, it can also be used for aching joints, muscle aches, menstrual cramps, nerve pain, headaches, constipation, and indigestion. Castor oil is the traditional choice for a compress because its composition remains stable as it penetrates the skin and enters the lymphatic system.

To detox the liver with a hot compress, saturate a thick pad (about ¼ inch or 5 millimeters) of cotton flannel or wool with castor oil. Carefully squeeze

Make a Liver Compress

1. Saturate a ¼-inch thick pad of cotton flannel or wool in castor oil.
2. Squeeze out any excess oil and lie down.
3. Place the pad over your liver on the upper right abdomen.
4. Place some plastic wrap over the pad.
5. Put a hot-water bottle or heating pad on top.
6. Leave in place for a minimum of 20 minutes.
7. Remove and wipe well with a dry towel.
8. Store the oily pad in a sealed plastic bag in the refrigerator for repeated use.

out any excess oil, because it can stain clothes and sheets. Lie down on a comfortable surface and place the compress over the liver, which can be found under the lower right ribs. Place some plastic wrap over the top of the compress and cover it with a hot-water bottle or heating pad for a minimum of 20 minutes or up to 1 hour. Keep the source of heat as warm as you can tolerate, refilling the hot-water bottle if necessary. Remove the compress and wipe your skin clean with a dry towel. You can store the oily pad in a sealed plastic bag in the refrigerator and reuse it up to a dozen times.

If you're not able to make a compress, simply place a hot-water bottle or heating pad over the liver to increase circulation. Electric heating pads are sometimes frowned upon because of the electromagnetic radiation they (or other electrical devices) produce. However, electric pads stay hot for a full session and are very convenient.

Wheatgrass Juice

Wheatgrass juice is one of the best liver cleansers I know. A standard dose is 2 ounces (60 milliliters) taken on an empty stomach twice daily. So drink up! Or consider a different method: wheatgrass is capable of detoxing the liver from either end of the intestinal tract. Serious wheatgrass users take rectal implants that shoot wheatgrass juice directly to the liver via the hepatic

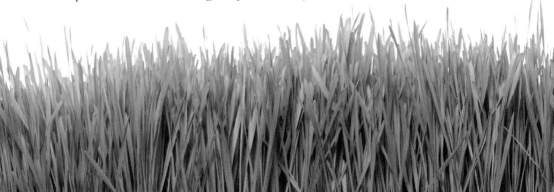

Ask Sproutman

Dear Sproutman: For ongoing health, can I include 2 ounces (60 milliliters) of frozen wheatgrass in the Grapefruit Liver Cleanser (page 111)? —*Julie*

Dear Julie: Wheatgrass juice is one of the best liver cleansers, and frozen wheatgrass juice is convenient to use. But I don't recommend mixing wheatgrass juice and the grapefruit drink. The Grapefruit Liver Cleanser works as a gentle cathartic for purging the liver and gallbladder; wheatgrass is more of a biochemical liver wash. Both promote slightly different processes, so use them at different times.

vein. The wheatgrass juice travels to the liver from veins in the sigmoid (lower) colon or the hepatic flexure further up. An implant involves squirting 2 ounces (60 milliliters) of wheatgrass juice using a bulb syringe (commonly available in pharmacies) into a pre-cleaned colon. Clean the colon with an enema prior to the implant, or the implant will trigger an evacuation and you'll need to repeat the process. Lie in the bathtub or on the bathroom floor and elevate your hips to help you retain the juice as long as possible; 5 to 15 minutes is typical.

Coffee enemas are also known for stimulating the liver, but wheatgrass delivers a wide range of phytochemicals that also scour and deepen detoxification. You can take wheatgrass implants daily, but just in case you find they're a pain in the butt(!), you can always drink wheatgrass juice instead. Although drinking the juice doesn't route it as directly to the liver as the implant, the drink is still a good cleanser.

THE INTESTINES

low is the key word to meditate on when trying to detox your intestines. That's why you'll use colon-cleansing drinks containing the gelatinous indigestible fiber from flaxseeds or psyllium seeds. Regular use of these drinks, along with a boost of milk of magnesia, will keep you regular and "in the flow."

Another ingredient that helps get the gunk out is bentonite clay. Like clay in general, bentonite clay is highly absorptive, and if you add the liquid form to your colon cleanser drink, it will turbocharge the drink's power. Because it's known for its capacity to absorb twenty times its weight in water, bentonite clay is extremely good at attracting pathogens and contaminants in the intes-

Cleanse Your Intestines with . . .

- colon cleansers using psyllium seeds or flaxseeds and bentonite clay
- milk of magnesia (page 7)
- activated charcoal tablets
- Vitamin C Flush (page 68)
- Water Flush (page 16)
- wheatgrass drink or rectal implant
- enemas or colon hydrotherapy

tines. Also, its negative ionic charge attracts positively charged toxins that cling to the particles of clay. Bentonite clay is commonly used for digestive problems, such as diarrhea and heartburn, but it must be used with care. Because it's capable of absorbing so much fluid, it could cause constipation (or in extreme cases, even dehydration) if misused. But you'll have no worries as long as you follow the recipe for Bentonite–Psyllium Seed Colon Cleanser (page 110).

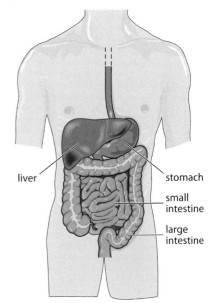

liver

stomach

small intestine

large intestine

Another product that does a good job of absorbing toxins is activated charcoal. It's probably most famous for its use in water filters, where it absorbs all types of organic compounds, such as pesticides and chlorine. But activated charcoal is also used medically as an antidote for poisons; in fact, it's so absorbent, it can interfere with medications. For our purposes, you can take it in tablet form, mostly to eliminate gas if you overeat during the transition back to solid food. You can also use activated charcoal tablets to treat diarrhea, indigestion, and flatulence.

Colon Hydrotherapy

The colon contains eight feet of plumbing that runs from your rectum to the cecum, a junction on your right side near the appendix that joins the colon to the small intestine. To do a deep cleaning, you can opt to have colon hydrotherapy, which is also known as a high colonic. A typical session consists of flushing your colon with 5 to 10 gallons (20 to 40 liters) of water over the course of one hour. You're assisted by a licensed colon hydrotherapist, but you're largely in control. This means that once the water tube is inserted in your bottom, you use your sphincter muscles to control the influx of water and also expel it as comfort dictates. The idea, of course, is to allow the water to gradually move up higher to the cecum so the entire colon gets flushed. The colon hydrotherapist is with you the whole time, coaching and massaging you to help you relax.

I recommend using milk of magnesia the night before your colonic appointment, so you can clear out a good bit of fecal matter before you go. That way, the time on the colonic table will be spent cleaning the higher regions of the colon. For the same reason, refrain from filling your stomach with water or juice before your session. You want your stomach to be as empty as possible, so you have the capacity to move the water around and flush the colon clean.

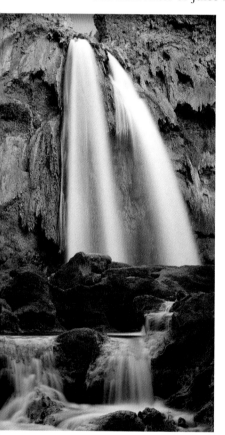

The primary discomfort you might feel during a colonic session is bloating, which persists until you release the flow of water. If you really want to get your colon clean, you'll need to tolerate both some massaging and some bloating. If you know this in advance, you can prepare yourself and achieve the maximum results.

Some people are concerned that a colonic will wash away the good bacteria from the colon, and it's true that lots of bacteria, both good and bad, are washed away in the wastewater. But given that 30 trillion bacteria inhabit a typical intestine, it's impossible to flush them all. The important issue is to control the balance between the good and bad bacteria, and cleaning house with a colonic is an opportunity to refresh that intestinal balance. Keep taking your daily probiotics, and the good bacteria will grow back quickly.

People have asked me whether it would be easier and less expensive to give themselves an enema instead of having a colonic. The difference between a colonic and an enema is the volume of water. An enema bag contains about 2 quarts (2 liters) of water. The process of taking an enema requires a certain amount of gymnastics. You have to stand up to fill the bag and lie down to install the enema tube with every bag of water you want to use. There are enema experts out there who have established rituals that include shortcuts and efficiencies, but for beginners, the process moves slowly and has a level of inconvenience.

Colonoscopies and the Dreaded Purge

If you've ever had the pleasure of getting a colonoscopy, you know that the blessed event requires you to show up with a clean colon so the doc can go sightseeing with his camera. To accomplish this, you're asked to drink a pharmaceutical purgative—something stronger than milk of magnesia or castor oil—the day before the exam. So you can expect to spend the day in the bathroom!

When I had my colonoscopy, I decided to skip the purgative and took a high colonic instead. But the doc made it known to me that one colonic was not enough. (Uh-oh!) It's really hard to flush out a colon perfectly in just one session. I learned that it requires at least two consecutive colonic sessions one day apart. Colonics are great, but they cost more than purgatives, and two sessions also take up a chunk of time. And although the purgatives may result in a tempestuous time on the toilet, a high colonic is not exactly your walk in the park either!

If you're due for some internal photography, you can make the choice: purgative or colonic. One consideration is to respect the doctor's protocol since it's in your best interest that he complete his task successfully. Purgatives also have the added benefit of flushing the entire intestinal tract, while a colonic is limited to the colon.

Whatever you decide, don't put off a regular colonoscopy; see resources, page 125, for a useful link that will provide more information about colonoscopies, such as how often they're recommended. Every year, 50,000 deaths are attributed to colon cancer. Colonoscopies can help doctors catch problems early enough to save lives. The topic still makes some people feel squeamish, but the benefits of colonoscopies are getting attention. Why not shed some light on this otherwise dark place? Many people know someone who has died from colon cancer. But no one has ever died from embarrassment.

A colonic takes about an hour, and the average enema takes at least forty-five minutes. A colonic cleans you with about ten times as much water as an enema, and it enables you to relax on your back and massage your abdomen. Finally, there's the advantage of having an assistant who is also a coach and masseur and takes care of the cleanup. In the end, a colonic is preferable as long as it fits into your budget. A session can cost from $60 to $100 in the United States. For more information on how to find colonic services, see resources, page 125.

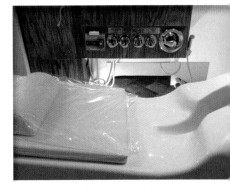

A modern colon hydrotherapy bench that allows the patient to regulate water flow.

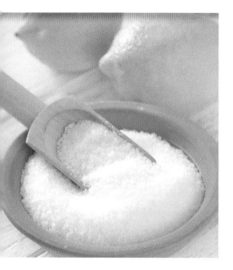

The Vitamin C Flush

Vitamin C is a potent detoxifying agent with a wide range of health and energy-boosting benefits. This flush uses vitamin C powder to trigger a bowel movement; at the same time, it will fulfill your daily requirement for vitamin C.

Use a buffered ascorbate powder, such as calcium or magnesium ascorbate. If you can, try to find a powder that combines potassium, calcium, magnesium, and zinc altogether (see resources, page 126). You'll be consuming more valuable minerals, and I prefer to get a balance of all of them rather than take just one or two.

Start first thing in the morning on an empty stomach. For the initial cleanse, make sure you have an open day until you learn how much time your body requires to purge. Stir 1 teaspoon (5 milliliters) of the powder into 6 ounces (180 milliliters) of water or divide that amount between water and juice. (My personal favorites are coconut water or prune juice.) Let the powder finish fizzing and then drink. This will be drink number one. Repeat the process, taking drink number two 15 minutes later. Keep repeating until you've had enough drinks to inspire a bowel movement. I like to make a batch of four drinks at a time. Then I can simply measure out a serving and keep the rest refrigerated in between.

Most folks require between 3 to 8 teaspoons (15 to 40 milliliters) of powder before getting a response. One teaspoon (5 milliliters) of powder typically contains 5 grams of vitamin C (check the label of your particular product to make sure), so most people experience the purge response after they've taken between 15 to 40 grams of vitamin C.

Use your diary to keep track of how many drinks, and therefore how many grams of vitamin C, it takes to flush your system. If you repeat this flush every few days or once per week, your notes will help you calculate how much vitamin C your body truly requires. That number is about 75 percent of what it took to initiate a purge. For example, if it usually takes 10 grams of vitamin C to initiate a purge, then theoretically your body absorbs and utilizes about 7.5 grams daily.

THE URINARY TRACT

etoxing the urinary tract is relatively simple during the Just Juice Diet, as so much of what you'll be doing for your digestive system, such as drinking juices and pure water, is also beneficial for the filters of your urinary tract: the kidneys. Keep in mind the important job the kidneys do and how juices play an important role in supporting the kidneys. Juices from celery, cucumbers, garlic, parsley, watermelon (with rind), and wheatgrass are particularly good for kidney health. In addition, corn silk, dandelion, hawthorn, juniper berries, parsley, and rose hips are famous herbal diuretics that can be taken as supplements or as tea.

Water is ultimately the best cleanser for the urinary tract, which is why I recommend that you drink at least 1 quart (1 liter) of the plain stuff daily! On page 17, you can read my discussion about which water is best. But for cleansing the kidneys, one type of water is ideal: distilled. Distilled water has no solids in it, no minerals, no electrolytes—it's laboratory pure. (Of course, most of us want minerals and electrolytes in our water, but that's another discussion). As far as the kidneys are concerned, distilled water means no work, and your "kids" are on vacation this week! Give them distilled water and they can kick back for a while before they have to go to work on the fresh juices.

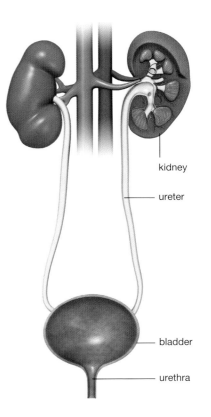

kidney

ureter

bladder

urethra

SPECIAL CARE FOR MOUTH, EARS, NOSE, AND EYES

Digestion begins in the mouth, so your mouth needs special attention the week of your fast. Indeed, at any time the state of your tongue and breath can indicate your level of intestinal toxicity. During your cleanse, the increased release of toxins will coat your tongue and teeth, so brush your teeth more frequently, scrape your tongue clean, and use a healthy mouthwash.

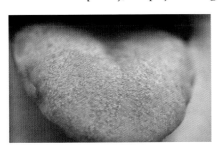

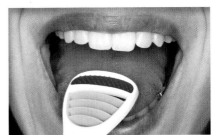

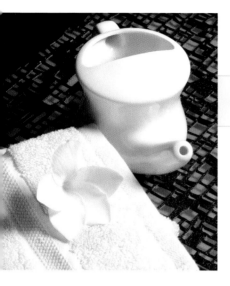

Tongue cleaning is actually another form of skin brushing; tongue scrapers are available at most natural food stores.

The state of your tongue and breath can indicate your level of intestinal toxicity.

Every orifice on your body, including your ears, nose, and eyes, can become an exit point for toxins. So if you notice earwax buildup, schmutz coming out of the corner of your eye, or unusual congestion, these symptoms can be attributed to your cleanse. Just a little extra attention is required: clean out the earwax, use some eyewash, or break out the neti pot for your nose.

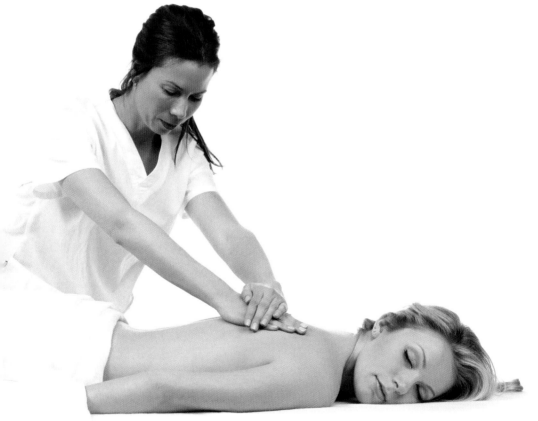

6

Transitioning Back to Solid Food

You've been eating all your life, so you know how to do it, right? Well, of course you do, but eating after a fast is different. Once the fasting part of the Just Juice Diet is over, you can't just dive back into your regular routine all at once. Good digestion depends on the secretion of enzymes from your digestive glands, pancreas, stomach, and liver. You turned off these valves during the juice fast, and there's no quick way to force them back on. Besides, you don't want to force them. You need a strategy for a gradual transition back to solid food.

How do you know when it's the right time to start eating? You may assume the right time is the day after the 7-Day Just Juice Diet concludes. After all, that fulfills the idea behind the name of the program, right? However, you may find yourself in a very good place after seven days of fasting, and you may not want to start eating again simply because it's the eighth day. That's okay. If you feel like you're on a roll, consider sticking with the fast for a few more days. Ten days is a very popular length of time for fasting. Longer fasts of twenty-one, thirty, or forty days require more mental and physical preparation and an open schedule.

Following a fast, most people are surprised to find how indifferent they are to food. However, your body will let you know when it's time to stop fasting. These questions might help you identify your readiness: Are you tempted by the food around you? Do you find yourself saying, "Wow, that looks delicious"? Or "I wish I could taste that!" These are indicators you should pay attention to during the transition back to food. (Just don't let these urges get a foothold during the first three days of just juice, when you need to resist your digestive system's hunger cues.)

The seventh day of the fast is a decision day. This is the time to exercise your intuition and examine your inclinations. If you have an urge to eat at this point, it must be genuine. On the other hand, if you remain impartial to the eating going on around you, pay attention to that too. Tune in and let your body guide you to prolong or conclude your fast.

Tune in and let your body guide you to prolong or conclude your fast.

GUIDELINES FOR RESTARTING DIGESTION

The return to eating solid food is sometimes the hardest part of the cleansing process. Why? I can sum it up in two words: discipline and temptation. To overcome these challenges, you need to follow a strict schedule.

After a seven-day fast, it takes at least three full days to build up the flow of your digestive enzymes. After a ten-day fast, it takes about five days. In general, your transition back to eating solid food should take about half the time you spent fasting, but there are variables. If you've always had a strong stomach, you may need slightly less than half the number of fasting days. However, if you have a weak digestive system, you may need slightly more time. In either case, don't push it. A rushed transition results in digestive distress, potentially including cramps, distension, gas, and a sour stomach. The stress resulting from an overly ambitious transition could ruin some of the health gains you achieved during the fast.

The three-day transition plan (Day 1, Day 2, and Day 3) described here is based on the 7-Day Just Juice Diet. If you extend your fast beyond seven days, think of your transition time not in terms of days but in terms of phases (Phase I, Phase II, and Phase III). Apply the following guidelines to each phase the same way you would to one day. Increase the time spent on each

Basic Guidelines for Restarting Digestion

Just as you did in the days leading up to your fast, plan your post-fast meals with care. I recommend the following:

- Continue to choose organics.
- Eat small portions.
- Eat frequent meals.
- Continue using probiotics.
- Plan for a transition time that equals half your fasting time.
- Maintain sufficient intestinal volume.

Probiotics for the Transition and Beyond

Continue taking probiotics throughout all phases of the transition back to solid food. In fact, I recommend that you continue using probiotics on an ongoing basis. Probiotics not only help restore colon health during cleansing, but they also play an important role in digestion, breaking down food and neutralizing waste over time. See page 25 for daily quantities and review recommended brands in resources, page 126.

phase so the total transition time equals half the time of your fast. For example, a ten-day fast requires five transition days, so the three phases would be spread over those five days.

TABLE 7. Return to solid food

TIME	SUGGESTED FOODS
Day 1 (phase I)	Juicy fruits (citrus, melons)
Day 2 (phase II)	Smoothies, simple soups
Day 3 (phase III)	Salads
Day 4 (phase IV)	All fruits and vegetables, nuts, and seeds
Day 5 (phase V)	Regular diet (or extend transition)

DAY 1 (PHASE I)

This is the first day of your transition back to solid food. If you're coming off a fast that lasted longer than seven days, consider this Phase I of your transition back to food.

Everything you eat on this first day must have a high water content, such as juicy fruits. Good examples are watermelons, cantaloupes, tomatoes, grapefruits, and oranges. Grapes and berries are acceptable as long as the skins are thin and you chew them well. Anything else you want to try that's juicy and not very fibrous is eligible. However, a fruit like an apple wouldn't be a good choice because it's very fibrous and not very watery. (Wait until Day 2, or Phase II, to enjoy apples.)

On Day 1 (Phase I), eat small, frequent meals and chew them very well. For example, have half a grapefruit, then finish the other half one hour later.

Small, hourly meals prime the pump that opens the digestive valves. This pattern teases your digestive glands, gently waking them up.

During Day 1, it's best to consume one food at a time. A whole meal might consist of a tomato or some watermelon, for example. Above all else, chew, chew, chew. Chewing is required to break down the fiber as much as possible to make food particles small and easier to digest.

> *Chew, chew, chew. Chewing is required to break down the fiber as much as possible to make food particles small and easier to digest.*

A great example of a small meal on this first day is a honeydew smoothie, which is very easy to make. Simply scoop out the flesh from a ripe honeydew melon and process it in a blender until smooth. Drink it in two or three sessions, so you don't take in too much at once. A smoothie like this provides about as much soluble fiber as a colon cleanser. However, because it's very watery, a honeydew smoothie won't overburden your digestive system.

Even though you're getting fiber from a simple smoothie, continue drinking the colon cleansers that contain flaxseeds or psyllium seeds (pages 108 to 110) on the first day after the fast and probably on the second day too. Colon cleansers are necessary because the portion sizes of the solid food you're eating are still too small to fill up your intestines. Your goal is to achieve some intestinal movement every day. Food that sits inside the intestines too long can age and ferment. By the third day, the volume of the solid food you take in should be sufficient to achieve that flow, so you can discontinue the colon-cleansing drinks at that time.

Also during Day 1, keep drinking the Grapefruit Liver Cleanser (page 111) and fresh green vegetable juice, but don't strain these items before drinking

Day 1 (Phase I) of the Transition

Here are the important points to remember on Day 1:

- Eat foods, such as juicy fruits, that contain a lot of water.
- Eat one type of food at a time.
- Make portions small.
- Chew thoroughly.
- Keep drinking fresh green vegetable juice.
- Stop straining juices, vegetable broths, and soups.
- Continue drinking colon cleansers.
- Continue using probiotics.
- Maintain your discipline and don't overload your system.

Foods for Day 1 (Phase I)

Try the following foods to slowly and gently restart digestion on Day 1:

- cantaloupe or honeydew melons
- citrus fruits
- grapes and berries with thin skins (chew well)
- leafy sprouts and baby greens
- tomatoes
- watermelon

them. If you've been using an external strainer on your juicer to filter out sediment, stop using it now. Drinking the small amount of sediment from your juice stimulates your glands, telling them to wake up and secrete. If you're drinking hot vegetable broth or any of the miso soups in the recipe chapter, you can stop straining those too. A little sediment helps open those valves!

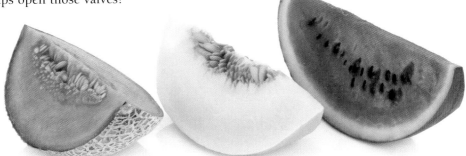

Bring On the Sprouts

Sprouts are an absolutely perfect food to use to break your fast—as long as they're green and leafy sprouts and not bean sprouts. Good examples are alfalfa, broccoli, buckwheat, clover, kale, radish, and sunflower. The water content of these baby leaves is similar to that of fruit, about 90 percent. But unlike fruit, sprouts are low in sugar and very easy to digest. Their cell walls are so tender, very little effort is needed to break down the fiber they contain. In fact, they practically melt in your mouth!

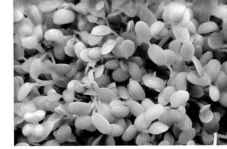

What? You don't have sprouts? As an alternative, try baby greens, such as kale, spinach, and mesclun mix. The leaves must be young and tender to qualify as a Day 1 food. Otherwise, stick to the sprouts

Use leafy green sprouts like these, but not bean sprouts.

during this first day and start the baby mesclun mix on the second day. Whatever you do, chew these foods extremely well and start with very small portions, such as ½ cup (125 milliliters) of sprouts or leaves. You can slowly expand portion sizes over the course of the day.

Beat Temptation

What if temptation gets the best of you and you overeat? If your stomach feels uneasy, sour, or you're getting cramps, here are a few suggestions:

- Lie down and place a hot-water bottle over your stomach.
- Take several deep breaths for a period of one minute.
- Walk briskly for ten minutes in fresh air.
- Try a dropperful of bitter herbs (page 81).
- Take supplemental digestive enzymes (see page 81).

These are all measures intended to compensate for your indiscretions. Of course, the best plan is to control your portion sizes and learn through experience how your body responds to small meals during the transition.

DAY 2 OR PHASE II

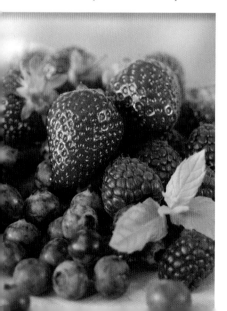

Any foods recommended for Day 1 (Phase I) may be included during Day 2 (Phase II). During this time, continue to thoroughly chew anything you put into your mouth. Break food down as much as possible with your teeth so your stomach will have an easier time. Continue to drink plenty of fluids to keep your intestines moving, but discontinue fresh juices if you want.

Now is the time to move beyond eating one single food at a time to combining multiple foods from a single family—for example, the citrus family, the melon family, the berry family, the stone fruits, and the tropical fruits. That means combining pineapple and orange, cantaloupe and honeydew, strawberries and blueberries, peaches and plums, mango and papaya . . . you get the idea. These food families go well together because, as far as your stomach is concerned, they require the same digestive enzymes.

During Day 2, you can begin to consume simple smoothies, but keep the initial portion size small, approximately 8 ounces (250 milliliters). Smoothies

TABLE 8. Sample menu for Day 2

TIME	SUGGESTED FOODS
8:00 a.m.	½ to 1 quart (500 milliliters to 1 liter) water
9:00 a.m.	Breakfast 1: Your choice of fruit; manage portion size carefully
11:00 a.m.	Breakfast 2: Another choice of fruit from the Day 2 list
12:30 p.m.	Lunch 1: Your choice of fruit, soup, smoothie, or greens
3:00 p.m.	Lunch 2: Your choice of fruit, soup, smoothie, or greens
4:00 p.m.	Your choice of liquids in between lunch and dinner or more fruit or greens
5:30 p.m.	Dinner 1: Your choice of fruit, soup, smoothie, or greens
7:30 p.m.	Dinner 2: Your choice of fruit, soup, smoothie, or greens
9:00 p.m.	Your choice of fruits or liquids
10:00 p.m.	Your choice of fruits or liquids

are not juices. If you put 2 bananas and 10 strawberries into the blender, mix them up, and drink them, you'll end up digesting all that food. Don't guzzle down a smoothie like you were your old self and expect your body to deal with it. Instead, sip your smoothie slowly. Make it with bananas, blueberries, and strawberries by following simple smoothie recipes, like those on pages 118 to 123.

If you eschew fruit smoothies because of their high natural sugar content, you can make green smoothies instead. These drinks can include many of the same greens you're eating in this early transition period, such as baby spinach, baby mesclun greens, and sprouts. See my recipes for the Basic Green Smoothie (page 118) and Energy Lifter Smoothie (page 119). Again, sip smoothies slowly and don't drink too much at one time.

Once you're able to drink at least 16 ounces (500 milliliters) of smoothies in a day, you can discontinue the colon-cleansing drinks. Because the fruit smoothies are a rich source of fiber, they ade-

Blend up berries to create a fruit smoothie. Add probiotic powder and stir it in.

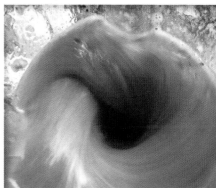

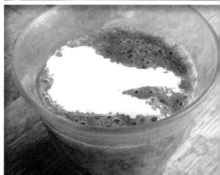

Day 2 (Phase II) of the Transition

Here are the important points to remember on Day 2:

- Continue eating foods, such as juicy fruits, that contain a lot of water.
- Eat meals that combine fruits from the same family.
- Drink simple fruit or green smoothies.
- Discontinue colon cleansers (optional) and fresh juices.
- Continue using probiotics.

quately replace the soluble fiber provided by the flaxseed and psyllium seed colon cleansers. Therefore, Day 2 is the first day you can transition from drinking the colon cleansers to drinking fruit and vegetable smoothies.

Nearly all fruits are eligible to go on your menu during Day 2 of the transition. Dried fruits and mature coconut (the big brown ones) are the exceptions. Dried fruits are too hard to digest at this stage because they're so concentrated. Plus, they're easy to overeat—all that sweetness packed into small morsels will be too much of a temptation. Instead, choose the fresh version of dried fruits you like. For example, if you love raisins, eat grapes; if you love dried pineapple rings, eat fresh pineapple.

Coconut is available in two different forms: brown and green. During the transition, choose green, or young, coconut because its meat is soft and watery like custard. Mature brown coconut has a very dry, fibrous meat that's high in fat and protein and more difficult to digest. Wait to eat mature coconut until you've fully graduated to eating solid food. In the meantime, enjoy young coconut as much as you desire, at any stage of the transition.

Self-Control

During Day 2, gradually begin to increase the volume of what you put in your mouth. Do this with the help of the brain in your stomach: the neuron

Foods for Day 2 (Phase II)

In addition to the foods approved for Day 1, try these foods to slowly and gently restart digestion:

- fruit (except dried fruit)
- fruit or vegetable smoothies
- miso soup with tofu and seaweed
- young coconut

sensors there provide a lot of information to the brain in your head about how your digestive system is doing. The stomach sends the head signals telling you to stop or slow down, but often there's a delayed response. You may find out twenty minutes after eating that you overdid it. Your stomach will feel sour and uneasy, and that's not what you want.

Once your glands start to wake up and your enzymes start to flow, it will become even more challenging to maintain your discipline. This is where self-control is critical. Manage the temptation! You're not up to full digestive strength yet. If you overdo it, compensate for any indiscretions by taking some bitter herbs (see page 81), digestive enzymes (see page 81), or other products recommended for handling excess (see page 81). Prevention is far better than treatment, however. Give your glands time to reboot: wait at least three days after a seven-day fast before returning to the portion sizes you used to eat.

That brings up a very good question: should you ever return to your previous portion sizes? That's up to you. This transition presents you with a wonderful opportunity to change your eating habits for good.

DAY 3 OR PHASE III

Any foods recommended for Day 1 or Day 2 may be included during Day 3 (Phase III). This is also the time when salads and homemade salad dressings can be added to your diet. Although you've enjoyed munching on sprouts and baby greens, your salad ingredients can now expand to include avocado, lettuce, olives, peppers, and my salad dressings (pages 94 and 95). Big, nutritious salads can replace green smoothies.

Day 3 is when you not only increase the quantity but also the complexity of what you consume. Gradual is the guiding theme here. Temptation will be strong. Once your taste buds wake up, you're instantly transported into a world of fabulous flavors and taste sensations, made all the more acute by their absence for the past week or more. You'll feel like you can eat anything—but you can't. This is arguably the most difficult of the three phases of transition because, as good as you feel, your capacity for digesting solid food has not fully returned. You are not *quite* your old self yet. You still can't consume *anything* you want in *any quantity* you want. (And by the way, you should, in general, erase that notion from your mind!)

Day 3 (Phase III) of the Transition

Here are the important points to remember on Day 3:

- Continue eating foods approved for Day 1 and Day 2.
- Expand your food choices.
- Start eating salads and homemade salad dressings.
- Gradually increase the volume and complexity of your meals.
- Discontinue smoothies if you prefer.
- Continue using probiotics.
- Maintain your discipline.

As you discovered during Day 2, there's a delayed response between consumption and feeling satisfied or even uncomfortably full. While eating, you may feel fine, but twenty to thirty minutes later, your stomach may start complaining. To avoid discomfort, keep these suggestions in mind: Avoid drinking water with your meal. Water and other drinks dilute your digestive enzymes, and you need them working at maximum concentration. Continue to chew thoroughly and pay attention to portion size. Use bitter herbs and digestive enzymes (see page 81) if necessary.

When you were fasting, your system was quiet and stable. Now, you've awoken the beast! You may find yourself temporarily feeling gaseous and

Food for Day 3 (Phase III)

In addition to the foods approved for Day 1 and Day 2, try adding the following foods now:

FRESH VEGGIES

- avocados
- celery
- cucumbers
- lettuce
- mesclun mix
- pickles
- olives
- olive oil
- peppers
- tomatoes
- sprouts

FRESH FRUITS

- apples
- bananas
- blueberries
- coconuts
- grapefruits
- grapes
- lemons
- mangoes
- pineapples
- raspberries
- strawberries

OTHER FOODS

- miso
- nori
- tamari
- tofu

crampy, particularly if you overdo it. Restimulating digestive enzymes takes time. If you've always had good digestion, then you'll likely find the transition back to solid foods easy, and your digestive strength will come back quickly. If you typically have digestive challenges, the speed of your transition and whether it will be a smooth or bumpy journey will depend on how judiciously you manage your intake.

Overcoming Temptation

The mantra you must practice during this transition is "discipline." Sometimes those devilishly seductive flavors lurking in your favorite foods launch a sneak attack, disabling all your rational thought and self-control. What are you going to do? Reach for this list of six techniques for combating overeating and stimulating your digestive resources.

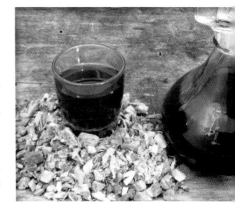

HERBAL BITTERS. A traditional European remedy, herbal bitters include cardamom, dandelion, ginger, fennel, and other bitter herbs that stimulate your pancreas, stomach, and liver to secrete enzymes. Take herbal bitters toward the end of your meals. There's a limited selection available on the market, but I do have some favorites that I recommend (see resources, page 126).

DIGESTIVE ENZYMES. Amylase, bromelain, cellulase, lipase, and papain are examples of digestive enzymes that you can take toward the end of meals. These supplements are helpful when your body is building up its production of your own digestive enzymes. (See resources, page 125.)

BARK CHEWS AND GUM. When chewed, cinnamon, licorice, and sarsaparilla stimulate the flow of saliva and gastric enzymes. I'm referring here to the real barks of plants, not powdered products. Cinnamon is famous for alleviating gas, nausea, and heartburn. Licorice bark is used to treat inflammatory bowel disease (such as ulcerative colitis), ulcers, and coughs. Sarsaparilla is not just the stuff of folklore but a genuine energizer and liver remedy. Even chewing mint gum, such as spearmint or peppermint, or whole fennel seeds effectively stimulates the flow of saliva and digestive enzymes.

HOT TEA. To quiet an uneasy stomach after dinner, drink hot tea. Chamomile, fennel, ginger, and peppermint teas are all soothing.

Products that Stimulate and Enhance Digestion

Need some help during the transition? Turn to the following:

- herbal bitters
- digestive enzymes
- bark chews and gum
- hot herbal teas
- probiotics
- exercises (deep breathing, walking outdoors)

PROBIOTICS. Don't forget probiotics, which help break down food and assist with the overall digestive process. Take them with the two largest meals of the day.

DEEP BREATHING AND EXERCISE. My favorite methods for reestablishing enzyme flow are deep breathing and exercise. For one minute before each meal, take slow, deep breaths; it's like adding oxygen to a fire. After the meal, take a brisk walk in fresh air. Walking keeps the digestive organs moving and the oxygen in your lungs flowing. Never lie down after a meal because it slows digestion. Do sit-ups, leg lifts, and inverted yoga postures between meals as part of your daily exercise regimen. These particular exercises will wake up your digestive glands.

DAY 4 OR PHASE IV

A t this point, based on a juice diet of seven days, you've completed the transition and can return to your regular diet. If you've extended your Just Juice Diet for longer than seven days, then this is your final phase. (For example, following a twenty-one-day juice diet, your return to a normal diet would occur ten days after you stopped juice fasting.) In either case, you're

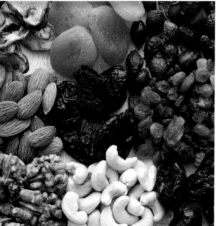

at a crossroads and can either return to your regular diet or choose a diet (see page 83) that continues to support cleansing.

If you just want to return to your original diet, your digestive system should now be ready for that. At this point, cleansing is over. The first foods I like to add back in are nuts, seeds, and dried fruits. These can include almonds, apricots, cashews, pumpkin seeds, raisins, and sunflower seeds, for example. Then begin to incorporate the foods you typically eat. Keep in mind that high-protein and high-fat foods, such as animal-based products, beans, dairy products, and grains initiate the switch from a catabolic (breaking down) phase to an anabolic (building up) cycle.

EXTEND YOUR DETOXIFICATION (PHASE V)

I f you have the discipline and the motivation, this is a perfect opportunity to extend the catabolic phase, or detox phase, of your diet. Here are some suggestions for adding an additional week of special regimens that continue your detox but incorporate more foods. Of course, you can choose to follow these eating patterns for much longer than one week; many folks follow these special diets on an ongoing basis—even for a lifetime. Following are some of the diets you could adopt to squeeze out an extra week or more of clean living:

RAW DIET. You've consumed a 100 percent raw diet during your cleanse and during your transition. Why not choose to maintain a raw diet for another week, but this time include nuts and seeds and dried fruits? Eating a raw diet means consuming nothing from a can or a box or anything that is cooked or processed. Here's the litmus test for raw foods: If it's in the same state it was when it was grown, you can eat that food. This includes foods that you can grow in your own kitchen—sprouts! Sprouts are energetically one step higher than raw foods in that they're "living foods" and maintain their life force right up to the moment you eat them.

VEGAN DIET. Your cleansing diet has also been vegan. How about going vegan for another week? This means eating no foods derived from animals. A vegan diet will give you more latitude than a raw diet, as it includes home-cooked and high-quality packaged foods.

GRAIN-FREE DIET. Staying grain-free is yet another option. Try eliminating all grains and flour products, including rice, oatmeal, bread, cookies, and so on. Starches can be the cause of a lot of internal congestion. You can be grain-free on either a raw or vegan diet.

GLUTEN-FREE DIET. A less strict version of the grain-free diet is the gluten-free diet, which allows grains such as non-GMO corn, millet, oats, quinoa, and rice. These foods don't contain a type of protein found in wheat (and related grains) that can irritate the digestive system. Eating a gluten-free diet means eliminating most commercial breads, bagels, pastas, and pizzas, which are omnipresent in conventional diets.

DAIRY-FREE DIET. Speaking of congestion, one of the biggest offenders is dairy. Humans are the only animals who drink milk after being weaned

Optional Diets for Extending Detoxification

Adopt one of the following diets, or a combination, to extend your transition or modify your long-term diet:

- raw (nothing cooked or processed)
- vegan (no animal-based foods)
- grain-free (nothing made of oats, rice, wheat, etc.)
- gluten-free (no wheat, oats)
- dairy-free (no milk or cheese)
- sugar-free

(let alone milk from another species!). In fact, a majority of people can't tolerate the lactose (milk sugar) in animal milk, so it comes as no surprise that dairy products are hard to digest and contribute to congestion. Vegans are dairy-free by definition, but you can be dairy-free on any diet. The longer you avoid dairy products, the more cleansing you'll experience. Choose non-dairy alternatives, such as almond, oat, rice, and soy milks and vegan cheese, instead of common dairy products. Experiment with different brands until you find your favorites.

SUGAR-FREE DIET. Going sugar-free is also very beneficial. Sugar is a primary contributor to metabolic syndrome, which includes pre-diabetes, obesity, and high blood pressure. The problem with sugar is prevalence and quantity;

Ask Sproutman

Dear Sproutman: I've heard that vegans can't get vitamin B_{12} from their diet and need to supplement. How can you recommend a deficient diet? —*Sandy*

Dear Sandy: It's true that vegans need to supplement with vitamin B_{12}, but so does everybody else! Our ability to absorb B_{12} diminishes as we age, even if it is in the diet, so everyone needs B_{12} supplements. These are commonly available as sublingual tablets that dissolve under the tongue. Animal-based foods provide B_{12} because animals make it inside their intestines. But guess what—we're animals too, and we also manufacture vitamin B_{12}. Since friendly bacteria are important in this process, keep taking probiotics and pile on fermented and bacteria-rich foods, such as miso, nondairy yogurt, nutritional yeast, pickles, sauerkraut, and tempeh, to name a few. Then dissolve that small B_{12} tablet under your tongue for health insurance and let the cows live.

Choose Organic Fruits and Vegetables

One important reason to choose organic fruits and vegetables is to avoid pesticides and other chemicals. Following are the lists of conventional produce that is most likely and least likely to be polluted and detrimental to your health.

FOODS HIGHEST IN PESTICIDES

- apples
- bell peppers
- celery
- cherries
- grapes
- lettuce
- nectarines
- peaches
- pears
- potatoes
- spinach
- strawberries

FOODS LOWEST IN PESTICIDES

- asparagus
- avocados
- bananas
- broccoli
- cabbage
- corn (fresh)
- kiwifruits
- mangoes
- onions
- papayas
- peas
- pineapples

Source: The Environmental Working Group, EWG.org

it's in almost all manufactured foods, and it's used in large amounts in sugary drinks. Added sugar can be a problem in homemade desserts too, because the quantities used in recipes are pretty high. Even natural sweeteners, such as agave nectar, honey, and maple syrup, can wreak havoc on the health of people who are inactive and overweight. Eliminating sugar for one week or longer after the 7-Day Just Juice Diet can contribute greatly to a cleaner, healthier you. A sugar-free diet allows you to enjoy naturally sweet foods, such as fruits and carrot juice, and pass on candy bars and sugar-sweetened breakfast flakes.

BUY ORGANIC FOR ONGOING DETOX

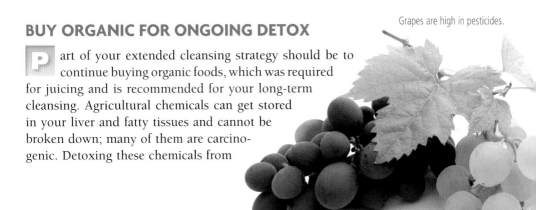

Grapes are high in pesticides.

Part of your extended cleansing strategy should be to continue buying organic foods, which was required for juicing and is recommended for your long-term cleansing. Agricultural chemicals can get stored in your liver and fatty tissues and cannot be broken down; many of them are carcinogenic. Detoxing these chemicals from your system is extremely difficult, so your best strategy is to avoid ingesting them in the first place.

In addition to being free of chemicals, organic foods are not genetically modified. Some researchers think that the increase in the number of GMO foods may be causing the significant rise in food sensitivities and allergies. GMO crops are banned or significantly restricted in thirty countries, including Australia, Japan, and the European Union. It could take decades to assess the impact of GMO crops on both our environment and our health. Don't take risks. Shop organic today—and always.

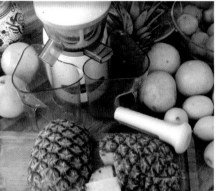

Pineapples are generally low in pesticides.

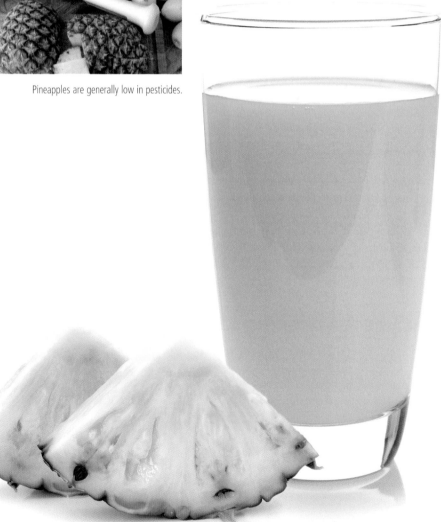

Fighting for Your Health

Detoxification is more important than nourishment. Maybe this sounds shocking, but you just survived seven days without eating and you feel better than ever! Why is that? In part, it's because you drank all those supernutritious juices! It's also because of the way your body is designed.

The lymphatic system transports twice as much fluid as the circulatory system. The former removes waste; the latter delivers nutrients. So, based on the way our bodies are designed, we should be focusing less on taking in food and more on removing waste. Yet our society is obsessed with food: We eat breakfast, lunch, and dinner. We snack in between meals, take coffee breaks, nibble while watching TV, and enjoy a little morsel (or more) just before bedtime. We're surrounded by food at restaurants, markets, grocery stores, and parties. We buy foods with dubious nutritional content from vending machines. And we're bombarded with food advertising. We're practically made to feel guilty if we're *not* thinking about food!

We've got our priorities backward. What's the result of this constant food intake? We've got neverending traffic jams inside our bodies! This congestion leads to infestation, infestation leads to infection, and infection leads to inflammation. Then we end up hurting. If inflammation goes on for years, normal cells degenerate under the stress and mutate. Mutation is the start of cancer. In an overwhelmed digestive system, even organic food can ferment and putrefy. Toxins that linger and fester in your tissues and glands can potentially surface decades later as disease.

PREVENTION TRUMPS TREATMENT

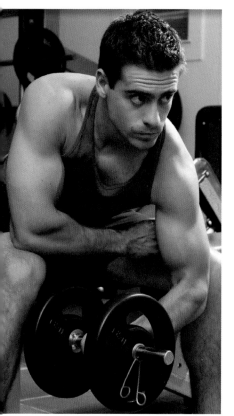

I like to think of the 7-Day Just Juice Diet as an investment in disease prevention. I fast this way a few times each year. For me, it's essential housecleaning. If I were to let the garbage pile up in my house, it would create infestation and disease. Detoxification requires taking the garbage out regularly. Periodically giving your body the opportunity to clean house puts you in a proactive mode that sharpens your body's defenses.

Most people don't have a prevention mind-set about their health. Instead, they spend time and money on enhancing their hair, eyebrows, skin, and nails. They quickly follow every new supplement fad that promises to magically cut pounds and increase energy. Our society's concept of a perfect body seems to be entirely external.

When I watch weight lifters push and pump, I admire how hard they work. Why can't we put that kind of effort into our internal health? Bodybuilders see results in a mirror. You can't see how much healthier your liver is after a fast. On the other hand, if you fail to work on prevention and detoxification, you may ultimately *feel* the effects of a sick liver. And ultimately, this will impact the quality of your days and the quantity of your years.

Sure, cleansing is hard work. Making all the drinks, fitting them into a schedule, doing the exercises, preparing an Epsom salt bath, getting a massage, and having a colonic—all of these take time and effort. But who else is going to make this effort for you? Certainly not the doctors. Spending seven days on just juice is good health insurance. Instead of spending money on medicine and doctors, you're spending it on vegetables. Starting today, I'm helping you open a "health and longevity bank account." This account is tax-free and disease-free. Every day, it builds your dividends of strength and immunity. This is the best investment of your life.

If you can't make the commitment to work on your health, how can you expect to conquer your illness?

Daily and Weekly Efforts for Ongoing Cleansing

Here are my recommendations for simple things you can do every day:

- drink fresh green vegetable juice
- drink Grapefruit Liver Cleanser (page 111)
- exercise daily; work up a sweat

Or set aside one day a week for doing the Just Juice Diet or devote a whole day to eating any one of the following nourishing and cleansing foods:

- fruits
- juices
- salads
- smoothies

REINVIGORATE YOUR CLEANSE: DAILY, WEEKLY, MONTHLY, YEARLY

A one-week cleanse can't erase decades of indiscretions. Detoxification is an ongoing process. Think how much cleaner your house is when you take care of it once a week instead of once a month. With a weekly cleaning, you can maintain and improve your home's appearance; but with only a monthly cleaning, you can't really keep up. Doesn't it makes perfect sense, then, that you need to do something daily, weekly, monthly, and annually to clean your body? Here are some suggestions.

Daily

If you can't make the commitment to work on your health, how can you expect to conquer your illness? Good health requires daily defense, and there are three things that I like to do every day to support ongoing detoxification.

First, I try to have fresh juice every day; for me, it's always fresh green vegetable juice. If I'm traveling, I'll get it from a juice bar. I don't generally recommend bottled juice, but there's a new alternative you can check out: brands that use high-pressure processing (HPP). Ultrahigh pressure is used to kill the yeasts, molds, and pathogens that end up in bottled juice. HPP sterilizes and extends the shelf life of the juice while leaving some vital factors intact. This juice is a step-up from pasteurized juice, but it's not a live or fresh product, no matter what the claim is on the label. So while I understand the need for convenience, opt for freshly squeezed juice whenever possible.

Second, I drink the Grapefruit Liver Cleanser (page 111) daily. It's easy to make, delicious, and very effective if taken on a regular basis.

And last but not least is physical exercise. Any aerobic or cardiovascular exercise that creates perspiration also supports ongoing detoxification.

Weekly

It would be great to routinely incorporate a special cleansing activity on the same day of every week. Committing to one activity one day per week adds up to fifty-two days of cleansing every year!

For example, you could choose to repeat the Just Juice Diet for one day each week. (You actually end up getting thirty-six hours of cleansing because a one-day fast stretches over two nights.) Alternatively, you could

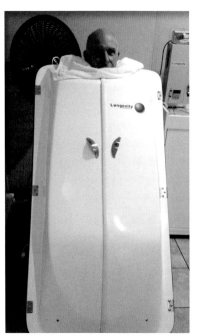

consume nothing but smoothies on one day or just eat fruit on one day. Perhaps switch things up: one week, have only smoothies for one day, and the next week, have only salads on that day.

Another option is to devote an entire day to colon cleansing. Make the Flaxseed or Psyllium Seed Colon Cleanser (pages 108 and 109) and drink it throughout the day, adding some milk of magnesia to help move things along. If you're so inclined, you could also do an enema.

Monthly

Any of the weekly routines could be done monthly instead. For example, juice fasting one day each month breaks bad habits and hits the restart button on your diet.

You also may want to consider scheduling one (or more) of the optional therapies that enhance detoxification each month. Getting a massage or

The author cooking inside an ozone sauna at 110 degrees F (44 degrees C).

other bodywork is great for squeezing out toxins. Soaking in a mineral bath or sweating in an ozone sauna at the local health spa is another good idea. Check out the different health offerings available near you and give yourself a monthly treat. Think of it as health insurance, not an expense.

Some people have asked me if it's wise to repeat the 7-Day Just Juice Diet every month. My answer is no; instead, I recommend doing the Just Juice Diet no more than once every three months. After seven or more days of fasting, your digestive system will go dormant and must reawaken. In between, your system requires an interval of restoration.

Your Regular Diet: Make It a Clean One

When you're not fasting, you can routinely take steps to improve your regular diet.

Reduce or eliminate:	Emphasize:	Shop:
• dairy products	• fruits and veggies	• at farmers' markets
• cooked fats	• salads	• for organic produce
• refined flour products		
• sugars and sweets		

Annually and Semiannually

Although you could do the 7-Day Just Juice Diet three or four times a year, once or twice yearly is the most popular option. Unless you are working on an intestinal condition, once or twice annually is also a good frequency for scheduling colonics.

My top recommendation for doing something yearly is to attend an annual health retreat. This is a vacation at a health-promoting location (preferably one that is beautiful and scenic!) where fresh foods, clean air, and sunshine are plentiful. You also could book a week at a health center where wheatgrass juice, raw foods, bodywork, and health treatments are offered.

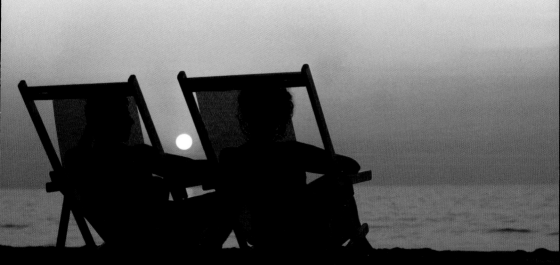

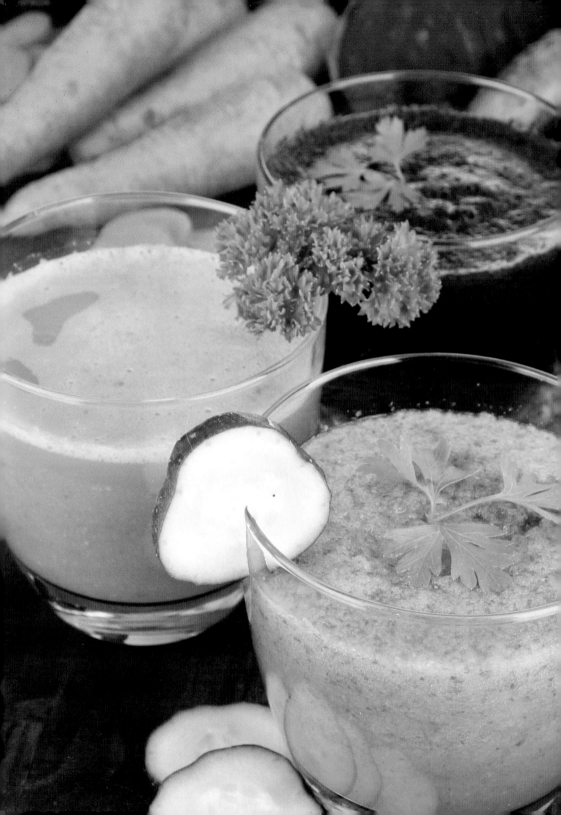

Recipes

I loved creating these recipes, but I don't believe that you need an exact recipe to make a great-tasting juice. In fact, my creative make-up is such that it's a struggle for me to even follow a recipe. When I juice, I use my senses, like an artist painting on a canvas. I put the bulkier veggies (greens, carrots, or apples) in first and then refine the flavors with the spicier ones at the end. I'm sure many people resonate with this approach. But I also realize that many other people appreciate having the structure of a good recipe, especially if they're new to juicing.

These recipes will provide guidance, but bear in mind that juicing by its very nature requires a little latitude. Vegetables vary in size and shape and the quantity of juice they produce (see page 28). So no matter what, there will always be a need for some wiggle room in juicing recipes.

For that reason, consider these recipes a starting point for your own experimentation and improvisation. Use your senses of sight, taste, and smell, as I do, to modify, explore, and deliver the perfect juice recipe for you. *Bon apétit!*

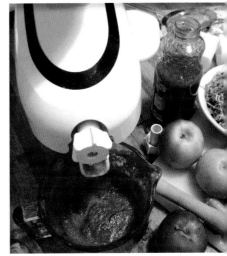

simple SALAD DRESSING

MAKES 7 TABLESPOONS (105 MILLILITERS), ENOUGH TO DRESS 2 CUPS OF SALAD

This recipe is easily doubled and leftovers can be stored in the refrigerator for up to five days.

¼ cup (60 milliliters) **extra–virgin olive oil**

2 tablespoons (30 milliliters) **freshly squeezed lemon juice** (about ½ lemon)

1 tablespoon (15 milliliters) **reduced-sodium tamari**

Combine all the ingredients in a small bowl or glass jar. Whisk until well combined or seal the jar and shake vigorously.

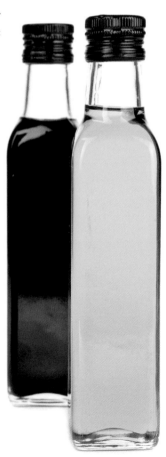

SIMPLE salad

A pre-fast salad can consist of everything on this list—or a big bowl of a single ingredient. The salty, fermented vegetables will add zest and interest.

VEGETABLE OPTIONS

avocado

bell peppers

celery

cucumber

greens (especially green sprouts, lettuce, spinach, kale)

olives

pickle

sauerkraut

sea vegetables (especially dulse, nori, kelp)

DRESSING

Simple Salad Dressing (page 94)

Select your choice of vegetables and the desired amounts. Slice into bite-sized pieces and combine in a bowl. Top with the amount of dressing desired and toss gently.

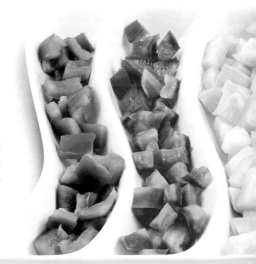

SIMPLE miso SOUP

MAKES ABOUT 1 CUP (250 MILLILITERS)

Miso is widely available in natural food stores or wherever Asian foods are sold. There are several varieties you can choose, ranging from strong to mild. I find white, mellow, or low-salt barley misos to be the mildest. You can also enjoy unstrained Miso Nori Broth (page 116) during the pre-fast.

2 tablespoons (30 milliliters) **white or other mild miso**

1 cup (250 milliliters) **hot** (but not boiling) **water**

1 teaspoon (5 milliliters) **grated onion** (optional)

Spoon the miso into a mug or small bowl. Add the hot water and stir until dissolved. Stir in the optional grated onion. Serve immediately.

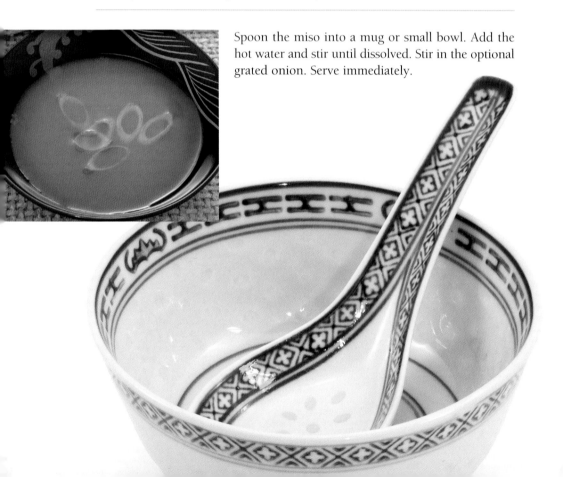

SPROUTMAN'S BASIC GREEN juice

MAKES ABOUT 2 CUPS (500 MILLILITERS)

This green juice recipe is used extensively in the 7-Day Just Juice Diet. You can easily double it to make your recommended daily quart (1 liter). The parsley and kale provide strong flavors, but the celery and lemon mellow the intensity. Most of the other green juice recipes in this section expand on this general formula. Use the milder recipes that follow if the flavor of this basic juice is too strong for you. However, it would be good to develop a taste for these greens as they're your best medicine.

4 stalks celery

15 to 20 sprigs parsley

15 stalks lacinato kale

2 tablespoons (30 milliliters) **freshly squeezed lemon juice** (about ½ lemon)

Juice half the celery, then half the parsley, then half the kale. Repeat in this order with the remaining vegetables. Stir in the lemon juice.

SPICY GREEN JUICE: Spice up the basic recipe with the addition of 1 to 2 teaspoons (5 to 10 milliliters) of reduced-sodium tamari, half a clove of fresh garlic, or ½ inch (10 millimeters) of fresh ginger. Add more to taste if desired.

MILD GREEN JUICE: If Basic Green Juice is too "green" tasting for you, add 1 to 2 cucumbers. Makes about 2½ cups (625 milliliters).

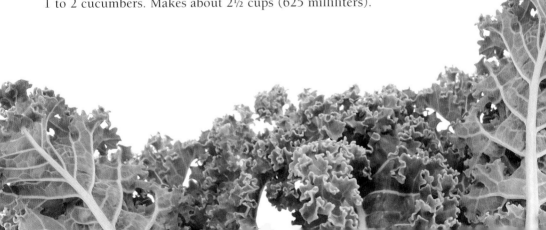

mild SPINACH JUICE

MAKES ABOUT 2½ CUPS (625 MILLILITERS)

Vegetables from the brassica family—broccoli, cabbage, collard greens, and kale—are loaded with healing compounds called glucosinolates, which can give these healthful veggies a slight medicinal taste. If you have trouble tolerating the intense green flavor of the Basic Green Juice, this recipe provides a gentler alternative by replacing the kale with spinach.

4 stalks celery

15 to 20 sprigs parsley

15 to 20 leaves spinach

1 to 2 cucumbers

2 tablespoons (30 milliliters) **freshly squeezed lemon juice** (about ½ lemon)

Juice half the celery, then half the parsley, half the spinach, and half the cucumbers. Repeat in this order with the remaining vegetables. Stir in the lemon juice.

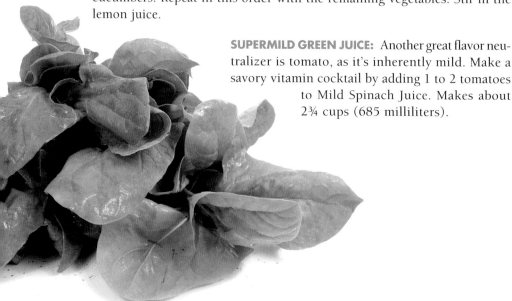

SUPERMILD GREEN JUICE: Another great flavor neutralizer is tomato, as it's inherently mild. Make a savory vitamin cocktail by adding 1 to 2 tomatoes to Mild Spinach Juice. Makes about 2¾ cups (685 milliliters).

TAMARI-GARLIC green JUICE

MAKES ABOUT 2 CUPS (500 MILLILITERS)

Juices are in effect liquid salads, and all salads go down a little easier with dressing. The combination of tamari, lemon, olive oil, and garlic adds the flavor of a salad dressing and pairs as well with juice ingredients as it would with a fresh salad.

---

4 stalks celery

---

15 to 20 sprigs parsley

---

15 stalks lacinato kale

---

1 to 2 cucumbers

½ clove garlic

---

2 tablespoons (30 milliliters) **freshly squeezed lemon juice** (about ½ lemon)

---

1 to 2 teaspoons (5 to 10 milliliters) **reduced-sodium tamari**

---

1 teaspoon (5 milliliters) **extra-virgin olive oil**

Juice half the celery, then half the parsley, then half the kale, then half the cucumbers, then all the garlic. Repeat in this order with the remaining vegetables. Stir in the lemon juice, tamari, and olive oil.

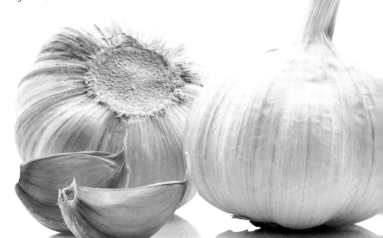

SPINACH-TOMATO juice

MAKES ABOUT 2½ CUPS (625 MILLILITERS)

This variation of Tamari-Garlic Green Juice (page 99) includes tomatoes and spinach to make a drinkable salad.

4 stalks celery

15 to 20 sprigs parsley

15 to 20 leaves spinach

1 to 2 tomatoes

2 tablespoons (30 milliliters) **freshly squeezed lemon juice** (about ½ lemon)

1 to 2 teaspoons (5 to 10 milliliters) **reduced-sodium tamari**

1 teaspoon (5 milliliters) **extra-virgin olive oil**

Juice half the celery, then half the parsley, then half the spinach, then half the tomatoes. Repeat in this order with the remaining vegetables. Stir in the lemon juice, tamari, and olive oil.

HOT TOMATO GREEN JUICE: Add some zest by including juicing an inch of poblano chile or your favorite hot chile, or simply add a pinch of cayenne.

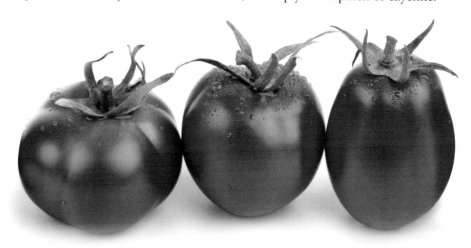

SPROUTMAN'S V-8 JUICE

MAKES ABOUT 3 CUPS (750 MILLILITERS)

Commercial "vegetable juice" is touted as being loaded with eight healthy vegetables, but it's really just tomato juice (which is why it's bright red) jazzed up with a smattering of other vegetables. Try making my version of this popular bottled juice and you'll notice a kaleidoscope of colors. In fact, the red from the tomatoes is barely visible.

4 stalks celery

15 to 20 sprigs parsley

15 stalks lacinato kale

1 to 2 cucumbers

1 to 2 tomatoes

½ clove garlic

2 tablespoons (30 milliliters) **freshly squeezed lemon juice** (about ½ lemon)

1 to 2 teaspoons (10 to 20 milliliters) **reduced-sodium tamari**

Juice half the celery, then half the parsley, half the kale, half the cucumbers, half the tomatoes, and all the garlic. Repeat in this order with the remaining vegetables. Stir in the lemon juice and tamari.

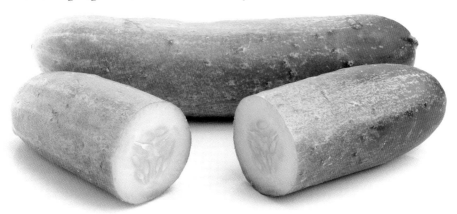

lemon-ginger GREEN JUICE

MAKES ABOUT 2 CUPS (500 MILLILITERS)

Ginger is best known for its sharp flavor, but behind that sharpness is a superstar in the world of plant medicine. Ginger is famous for helping with digestion and metabolism, but it's also an anti-inflammatory. If you're not used to eating fresh ginger, start with a little bit and work your way up to the amount suggested here. Ginger can make your juice taste spicy hot, but the more of it you can tolerate the better. Be sure to add the ginger in the middle of the juicing process so it gets fully squeezed.

4 stalks celery

15 to 20 sprigs parsley

15 stalks lacinato kale

½ inch (10 milliliters) **fresh ginger**

2 tablespoons (30 milliliters) **freshly squeezed lemon juice** (about ½ lemon)

Juice half the celery, then half the parsley, half the kale, and all the ginger. Repeat in this order with the remaining vegetables. Stir in the fresh lemon juice.

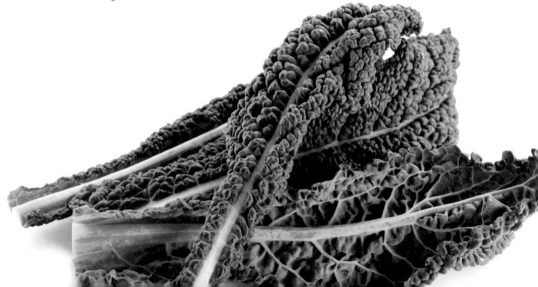

CARROT spinato JUICE

MAKES 2 CUPS (500 MILLILITERS)

Spinach and garlic always remind me of Italian food. For this juice, choose carrots that aren't very thick so they'll slide down the feed chute effortlessly.

10 carrots

2 cucumbers

15 to 20 leaves spinach

½ clove garlic

Juice half the carrots, then half the cucumbers, half the spinach, and all the garlic. Repeat in this order with the remaining vegetables.

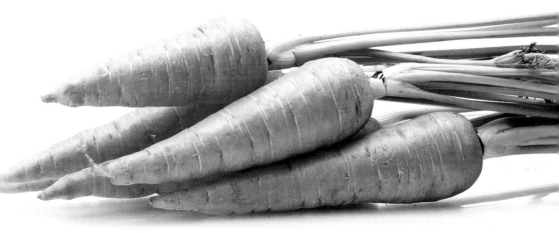

granny's GREEN JUICE

MAKES 2 CUPS (500 MILLILITERS)

This is a treat to make when the first Granny Smith apples of the season appear. The combination of cucumber and ginger will quench your thirst and put zip in your step.

3 cucumbers

15 to 20 leaves spinach

1 Granny Smith or other tart, juicy apple

½ inch (10 milliliters) **fresh ginger**

Juice half the cucumbers, then half the spinach, half the apple, and all the ginger. Repeat in this order with the remaining ingredients.

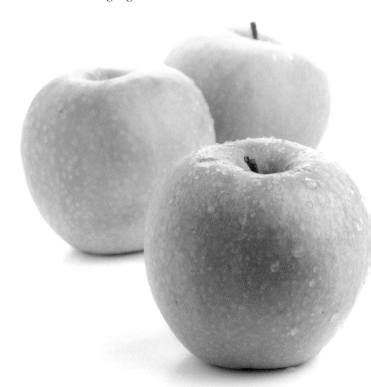

sweet BEET JUICE

MAKES ABOUT 2 CUPS (500 MILLILITERS)

Sweet juices are great for whenever you need a pick-me-up, and the rich color of this juice is sure to put a smile on your face.

7 to 10 carrots

1 beet

1 Granny Smith or other tart, juicy apple

Juice half the carrots, then half the beet, then half apple. Repeat in this order with the remaining ingredients.

SWEET AND ZINGY BEET JUICE: Include ½ inch (10 millimeters) fresh ginger, adding all of it between the first juicing of the carrots and beet so it will be fully squeezed.

SWEET CUCUMBER JUICE: Replace the beet with 1 to 2 cucumbers.

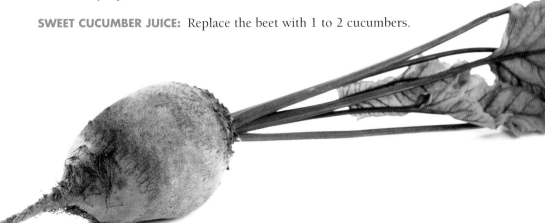

PINEAPPLE-APPLE *juice*

MAKES ABOUT 4 CUPS (1 LITER)

Pineapple is easier to juice than you might think. No peeling is necessary! Sadly, not all juicers can process pineapple's sinuous pulp. If your machine clogs, try using smaller pieces. It also helps to alternate pineapple with a firm fruit, such as a hard apple.

1 pineapple

2 Granny Smith or other tart, juicy apples

Remove the crown of the pineapple and rinse the pineapple clean. You may also want to cut out the bottom core, because it's very hard and dry and produces little juice. Slice the unpeeled pineapple into pieces that will fit into the chute of your juicer. Alternate between juicing pieces of pineapple and pieces of apple.

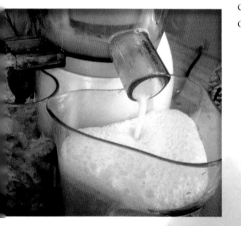

Although these recipes call for prune juice or coconut water, these are only suggestions. Choose your favorite bottled juice. Personally, I don't enjoy tomato or citrus with a mucilage, but almost any other fruit juice—such as apple, mango, cherry, grape, papaya, pear, or pomegranate—will work well. (Note: Some of these may need to be strained.) You can also use herbal teas, aloe vera juice, kombucha, unsweetened nut or grain milks, and even sauerkraut juice or pickle juice. Keep in mind that you'll be mixing these juices with equal amounts of water to reduce their sugar content. Unlike fresh-squeezed juice, colon-cleansing drinks don't require refrigeration, especially if you drink them the day they were made.

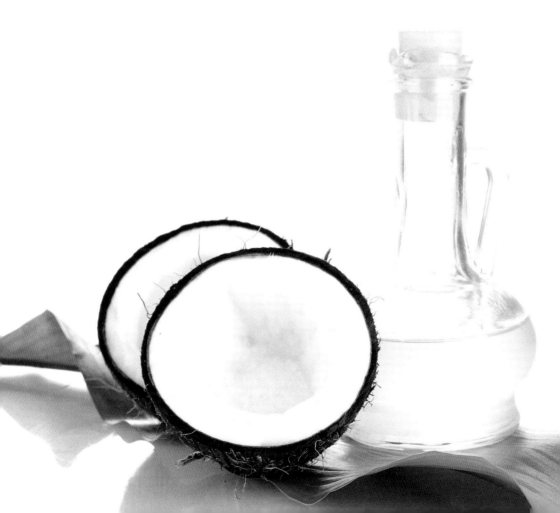

flaxseed COLON CLEANSER

MAKES 1 QUART (1 LITER)

Many people like to use flaxseed meal in a colon-cleansing drink because flaxseeds impart a pleasant nutty flavor. The only downside to doing this is that flaxseed meal is generally very coarsely ground. The coarse shells in the meal result in a good deal of insoluble fiber, similar to bran. If possible, look for ground flaxseeds that are as finely milled as flour. Either brown or blond flaxseeds are fine to use. If you have a blender with a tapered-bottom jar, you can grind whole flaxseeds yourself, and you'll have the benefit of knowing the meal is fresh. Just make sure the end result is as fine as flour.

2 cups (500 milliliters) **prune juice or coconut water**

2 cups (500 milliliters) **water**

½ cup (125 milliliters) **finely milled flaxseed meal**

Combine all the ingredients in a blender and process for 15 seconds. Let the mixture sit for 5 minutes, then process again for 15 seconds. The consistency should be like a thick shake but not so thick that it would be unappealing to drink. Divide the mixture between two drinking bottles.

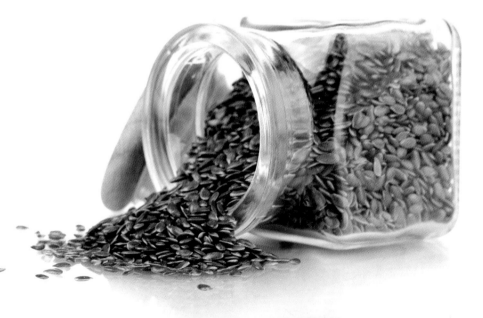

PSYLLIUM SEED COLON cleanser

MAKES ABOUT 1 QUART (1 LITER)

2½ cups (625 milliliters) **water**

1 cup (250 milliliters) **plain unsweetened nondairy milk**

½ cup (125 milliliters) **prune juice or coconut water**

3 tablespoons (45 milliliters) **psyllium seed husk powder**

Combine all the ingredients in a blender and process for 15 seconds. Let the mixture sit for 5 minutes, then process again for 15 seconds. The consistency should be like a thick shake but not so thick that it would be unappealing to drink. Divide the mixture between two drinking bottles. (See pages 6 and 47.)

Ask Sproutman

Dear Sproutman: I was just wondering whether nut milks or soy milk are okay to drink on a fast. —*Laurie*

Dear Laurie: Yes, nut milks and soy milk are excellent for the colon-cleanser drinks. Otherwise, only drink them in moderation, maybe once per day. Commercial nut and grain milks are all pasteurized, so homemade nondairy milks would be better. But commercial nut milks are widely available and convenient. Read the labels to make sure they don't contain added sugars or preservatives.

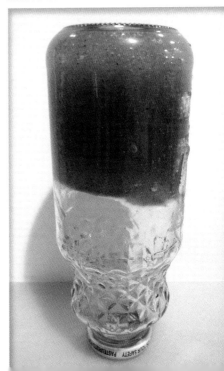

Oops! This is what happens when the psyllium mixture is too thick!

BENTONITE–PSYLLIUM seed COLON CLEANSER

MAKES 1 QUART (1 LITER)

The absorption ability of bentonite clay gives this cleanser a lot of grabbing power (see page 64). Always dilute bentonite clay in water with psyllium seeds, as in this recipe.

2½ cups (625 milliliters) **water**

1 cup (250 milliliters) **plain unsweetened nondairy milk**

¼ cup (60 milliliters) **prune juice or coconut water**

3 tablespoons (45 milliliters) **psyllium seed husk powder**

2 tablespoons (30 milliliters) **liquid bentonite clay**

Combine all the ingredients in a blender and process for 15 seconds. Let the mixture sit for 5 minutes, then process again for 15 seconds. The consistency should be like a thick shake but not so thick that it would be unappealing to drink. Divide the mixture between two drinking bottles.

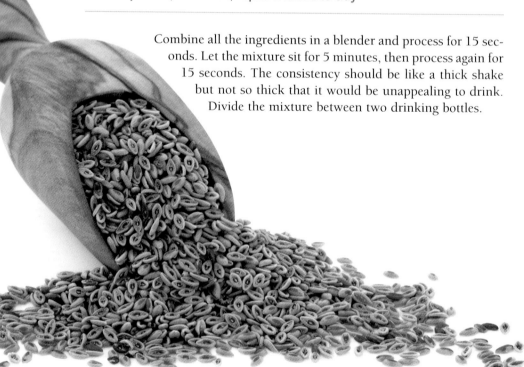

grapefruit LIVER CLEANSER

MAKES ABOUT 1 CUP (250 MILLILITERS)

This recipe stimulates the liver and gallbladder, encouraging a gentle purge of those two glands. The oil in this recipe is such a small amount that it's only enough to stimulate the gallbladder and activate its functioning but not burden it. For more information on liver cleansing, see page 60.

1 pink or white grapefruit

2 tablespoons (30 milliliters) **freshly squeezed lemon juice** (about ½ lemon)

1 teaspoon (5 milliliters) **extra-virgin olive oil**

½ clove garlic, pressed (optional)

Juice the grapefruit and lemon using an electric or hand-operated citrus juicer. Pour through a fine-mesh sieve to strain out the pulp. Combine the juices with the oil and the optional garlic.

NOTE: I recommend an electric citrus juicer over a manual one to extract the grapefruit and lemon juice because it's more convenient, especially since you'll make this drink daily. Lemon juice keeps well in the refrigerator, so juicing lemons in advance is also a time-saver. I juice about four lemons at a time (which makes one cup) and store the juice in the refrigerator for daily use. Strain out the pulp as best you can.

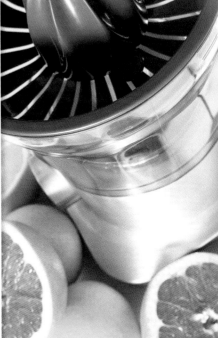

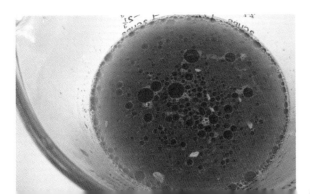

APPLE CIDER VINEGAR drink

MAKES ABOUT 1 CUP (250 MILLILITERS)

This ancient folk remedy and general tonic is a superb drink that's easy to make and doesn't require a juicer. Choose a quality brand of apple cider vinegar, one that clearly contains some sediment (known as the "mother") on the bottom of the bottle. You can make this drink stronger or lighter by adjusting the amount of vinegar or sweetener. This recipe is traditionally made with honey, but you can use maple syrup, agave nectar, stevia, or another sweetener instead.

1 to 2 teaspoons (5 to 10 milliliters) **apple cider vinegar**

1 cup (250 milliliters) **water**

1 teaspoon (5 milliliters) **honey or other sweetener**

Pour all the ingredients into a glass jar. Seal tightly and shake until combined. Drink immediately or store in the refrigerator for up to 2 days.

Benefits of Apple Cider Vinegar

Apple cider vinegar is purported to treat a wide variety of conditions, from removing warts to reversing aging! But you'll be interested to know it can help you lose weight, curb your appetite, and detoxify. Researchers in Japan measured decreases in body mass index, waist circumference, and serum triglycerides when people included vinegar in their daily diet. At the Department of Nutrition at Arizona State University, researchers were able to lower the blood glucose levels of diabetics by giving them only 2 tablespoons (30 milliliters) of vinegar at bedtime. Finally, at the Central Research Institute in Japan, rats fed vinegar excreted more bile acids, improved body detox- ification, and reduced their body fat by 10 percent. Apple cider vinegar is on your list of optional drinks—enjoy it!

HOT lemon TEA

MAKES ABOUT 1 CUP (250 MILLILITERS)

This is an easy drink to make when you're in the mood for something hot, and it's also cleansing for your liver. I've been asked about the acid in the lemon tea eating away tooth enamel. Although this is unlikely, if you have any concerns, you can always rinse your mouth with either plain water or a glass of water with ½ teaspoon (2.5 milliliters) of baking soda mixed into it.

1 tablespoon (15 milliliters) **freshly squeezed lemon juice**

1 cup (250 milliliters) **hot water**

1 teaspoon (5 milliliters) **extra-virgin olive oil**

1 clove garlic, pressed (optional)

Pour the lemon juice through a fine-mesh sieve to strain out the pulp. Add the water, oil, and optional garlic to the lemon juice and stir to combine. Drink immediately.

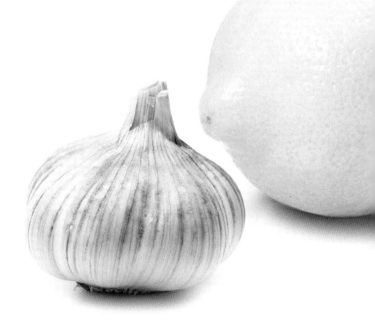

HOT ginger TEA

MAKES ABOUT 1 CUP (250 MILLILITERS)

You can make a double serving of this, drink half of it right away, and let the other half steep even longer while it cools. Once cold, refrigerate the extra serving in a jar and reheat it when you feel like having ginger tea again.

1 teaspoon (5 milliliters) **grated fresh ginger**

1 cup (250 milliliters) **hot water**

1 tablespoon (15 milliliters) **freshly squeezed lemon juice**

Stir the ginger into the water. Let steep for 5 to 10 minutes. Stir in the lemon juice. Pour through a fine-mesh sieve to strain out the ginger and lemon pulp. Drink immediately.

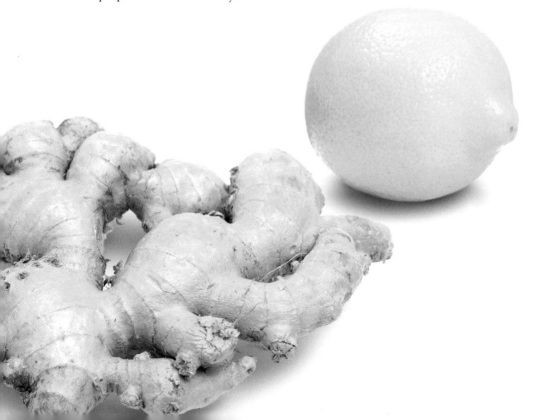

INSTANT VEGETABLE broth

MAKES ABOUT 1 CUP (250 MILLILITERS)

Hot broth can be a satisfying break from a cold juice diet. Making hot broth with broth powder is as fast as making a cup of tea. There are several good vegan broth powders and even liquid broth you can buy (see page 127). Just make sure they're gluten-free, flour-free, vegan, and contain no preservatives, genetically modified ingredients, or artificial flavors or colors.

1 cup (250 milliliters) **water**

1 tablespoon (15 milliliters) **vegan broth powder**

Combine the water and broth powder in a small saucepan. Simmer over medium-high heat for 5 minutes. Pour through a fine-mesh sieve to strain out any sediment. Drink immediately.

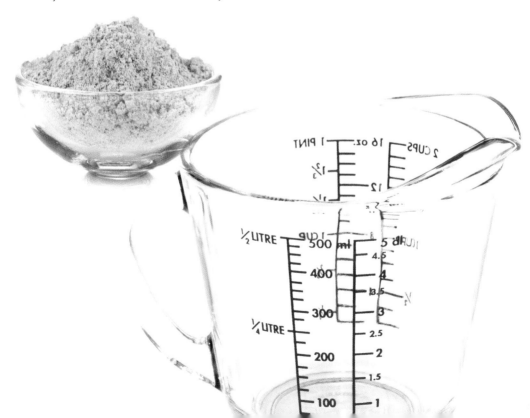

MISO nori BROTH

Although you can use any type of miso for this recipe, I favor the mild varieties, such as barley miso, white miso, or mellow miso. Using a blender to combine these ingredients reduces the number of steps and utensils you'll need.

1 cup (250 milliliters) **water**

One ¼-inch (5 millimeters) **slice onion, cut into quarters and finely chopped**

1 sheet nori

1 to 2 tablespoons (15 to 30 milliliters) **white or mild miso**

Put the water and onion in a small saucepan. Crumble in the nori. Alternatively, process the water, onion, and nori in a blender for 10 seconds, then pour into a small saucepan. Simmer over medium-high heat for 5 minutes. Remove from the heat and let cool for 1 minute. Add the miso and stir until dissolved. Pour through a fine-mesh sieve to strain out the solids.

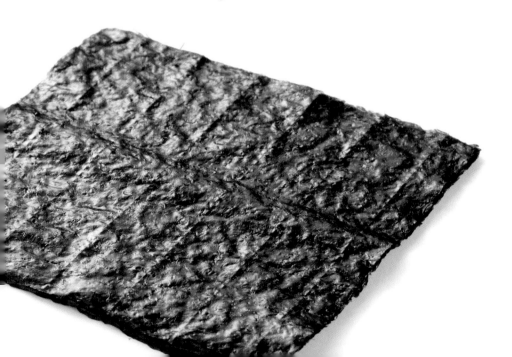

homemade VEGETABLE BROTH

MAKES 4 QUARTS (4 LITERS)

Homemade broth involves a fair amount of prep work, which is why I recommend instant broth powders most of the time. I would rather see you spend your time using your juicer or going to a health spa for a massage. If you're lucky enough to have Grandma or Mom living nearby, and they happen to be old-school connoisseurs, ask them to make some homemade broth for you. Almost any vegetables can be used to make broth, although cabbage, broccoli, and any other strongly flavored vegetables in the brassica family can be overpowering.

3 quarts (3 liters) water

1 large onion, chopped

1 leek, thinly sliced

3 cloves garlic, grated or pressed

2 to 3 carrots, chopped

2 parsnips, chopped

2 to 3 stalks celery, chopped

15 sprigs parsley, chopped

2 teaspoons (10 milliliters) sea salt, Celtic salt, or Himalayan salt

Pour the water into a large stockpot and bring to a boil over high heat. Add the remaining ingredients and return to a boil. Decrease the heat to low, cover, and simmer until the vegetables are very soft, 45 to 60 minutes. Let cool. Pour through a fine-mesh sieve to strain out all solids. Pour into one-quart jars and store in the refrigerator for 3 to 4 days.

Ask Sproutman

Dear Sproutman: Can you use the pulp that's left after juicing vegetables to make homemade broth? —*Cheryl*

Dear Cheryl: The different juice combinations I recommend are designed for juice flavors, and their pulp proportions are not necessarily well suited for broth. Nevertheless, it's a great idea and would be a worthwhile experiment!

BASIC GREEN smoothie

MAKES ABOUT 2½ CUPS (625 MILLILITERS)

If the flavor of the greens in this drink is too much for you, neutralize it by adding more tomato or a peeled cucumber. Note that baby spinach and baby kale are smaller and more delicate than their mature counterparts.

1¼ cup (310 milliliters) **chopped tomato**

¾ cup (180 milliliters) **chopped fresh parsley**

1½ cups (375 milliliters) **baby spinach or kale, firmly packed**

2 to 3 tablespoons (30 to 45 milliliters) **freshly squeezed lemon juice** (about 1 lemon)

1 teaspoon (5 milliliters) **extra-virgin olive oil**

1 to 2 teaspoons (5 to 10 milliliters) **reduced-sodium tamari**

½ cup **water, as needed**

Put the tomato, parsley, spinach, lemon juice, olive oil, and tamari in a blender and pulse until smooth. Add just enough water, 1 tablespoon at a time, as needed to achieve a drinkable consistency. Drink immediately or pour into storage bottles and store in the refrigerator for up to 2 days.

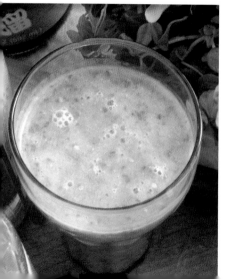

energy lifter SMOOTHIE

MAKES ABOUT 2 CUPS (500 MILLILITERS)

This drink is actually a delicious, blended raw soup—rich, satisfying, and energizing.

¼ cup (60 milliliters) **dulse**

1 cup (250 milliliters) **baby lettuce or sunflower sprouts**

½ **avocado, peeled**

½ **Granny Smith apple, chopped, or** ¼ cup (60 milliliters) **freshly squeezed lemon juice** (about 1 lemon)

½ cup (125 milliliters) **water, plus more if needed**

3 to 6 sprigs parsley, chopped

½ small clove garlic

Pinch cayenne

Soak the dulse in enough water to cover for 10 minutes. Drain. Put the dulse and the remaining ingredients in a blender and process until smooth. Add more water if needed to achieve a smooth but not-too-thick consistency. Drink immediately or pour into storage bottles and store in the refrigerator for up to 2 days.

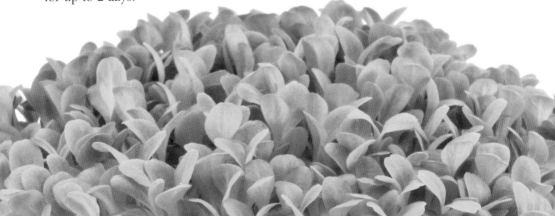

ANTIOXIDANT fruit SMOOTHIE

MAKES ABOUT 2 CUPS (500 MILLILITERS)

Frozen organic fruits are a convenient alternative for this recipe. They're available any time of year, and you can use only what you need and return the rest to the freezer. Leave at least an hour between drinking a fruit smoothie like this one and a green smoothie. The latter is mostly vegetables, and fruits and vegetables digest at different rates.

1 banana, chopped

½ cup (125 milliliters) **water, plus more if needed**

1 cup (250 milliliters) **large strawberry halves or whole small strawberries**

½ cup (125 milliliters) **blueberries**

1 to 2 teaspoons (5 to 10 milliliters) **probiotic powder**

Put the banana and water in a blender and process until smooth and thick, like a milkshake. Add the strawberries and blueberries and process again, adding additional water as needed to obtain a thick, smooth consistency. Add the probiotic powder and process briefly. Alternatively, pour the mixture into a glass and stir in the powder. Drink immediately or pour into storage bottles and store in the refrigerator for up to 2 days.

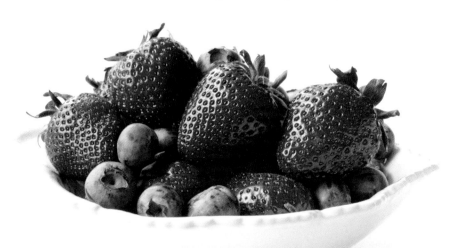

Other Fruit Smoothie Options

You can use any of your favorite fruits to make smoothies, but keep it simple. Don't use more than four fruits in a mixture because fewer varieties will be easier to digest. I like to mix bananas with apples, peaches, papaya, or berries. Add only enough water for the fruit to move easily in the blender so you can achieve a thick, shake-like consistency.

Frozen bananas are a great addition to fruit smoothies. They chill the mixture immediately and make the smoothie thicker than fresh bananas. If you have more fresh bananas than you can keep up with, peel them, wrap them individually in wax paper, and freeze them. Alternatively, chop them up and store them in a ziplock freezer bag or plastic container. That way they'll be easy to add to the blender.

If you're digesting solid food well at this point, you might opt to increase the complexity of your smoothies by adding supplement powders, such as nutritional yeast, wheatgrass powder, or probiotic powder. Add a little more water if necessary, just enough so the smoothie will still be thick but can move easily in the blender, creating a whirlpool as it spins.

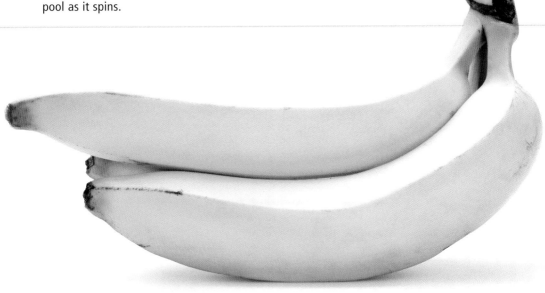

cantaloupe SMOOTHIE

MAKES ABOUT 2 CUPS (500 MILLILITERS)

Cantaloupe makes a sweet, rich-tasting smoothie. It doesn't get simpler than this!

½ cantaloupe, peeled and cut into chunks

¼ cup (60 milliliters) **water, plus more if needed**

Put the cantaloupe and water in a blender and process until smooth and thick. Add more water if needed to facilitate blending, but use only enough to create a whirlpool in the blender. Drink immediately or pour into storage bottles and store in the refrigerator for up to 2 days.

MELON SMOOTHIE: Replace the cantaloupe with another type of melon, but avoid watermelon because of the seeds that are distributed throughout the flesh.

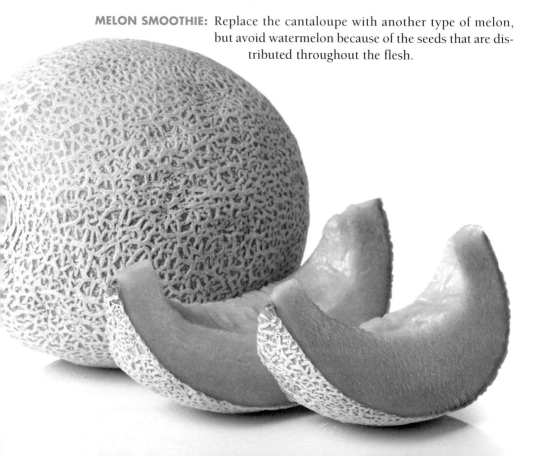

OAT MILK–PAPAYA smoothie

MAKES ABOUT 2 CUPS (500 MILLILITERS)

Oat milk or your favorite nondairy milk can be a very satisfying coming-off-a-fast drink, and it's a great addition to smoothies. You can use a commercial brand or one that you've made at home. No papaya? Feel free to substitute with peaches or apples. Nutritional yeast is a tasty inactive food yeast, rich in B vitamins, that can be added to any smoothie.

1 cup (250 milliliters) **commercial oat milk or strained Homemade Oat Milk** (page 124)

½ cup (125 milliliters) **water, plus more if needed**

½ ripe papaya, peeled, seeded, and chopped

2 tablespoons (30 milliliters) **oat bran**

1 tablespoon (15 milliliters) **nutritional yeast**

Put all the ingredients in a blender and process until smooth. Add more water if needed to achieve a smooth but not-too-thick consistency. Drink immediately or pour into storage bottles and store in the refrigerator for up to 2 days.

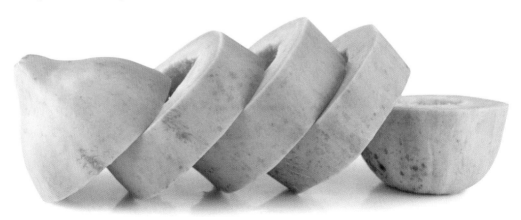

homemade OAT MILK

MAKES ABOUT 3 CUPS (750 MILLILITERS)

It's easy to make your own oat milk. The basic recipe is incredibly simple, with just a couple of ingredients. If you want a thicker milk, use less water and press the pulp more than once. You can also thicken it by cooking the oats before blending them. I'll leave that up to you, but the beauty of this recipe is that it's raw.

---

1 cup (250 milliliters) **organic rolled oats**

---

3 cups (750 milliliters) **water**

---

1 to 2 tablespoons (15 to 30 milliliters) **maple syrup or other sweetener**

Soak oats in water to cover for at least 10 minutes (soak them longer if a thicker milk is desired). Drain the soaking water and put the oats in a blender with the water and maple syrup. Process until smooth and creamy.

If you're fasting, remove the sediment by pouring the milk through a fine-mesh sieve or a strainer lined with cheesecloth. Stir and squeeze the pulp as the milk drains. If you're not fasting, you can leave in the sediment if you like.

Refrigerate and drink within 3 to 5 days. Shake before using.

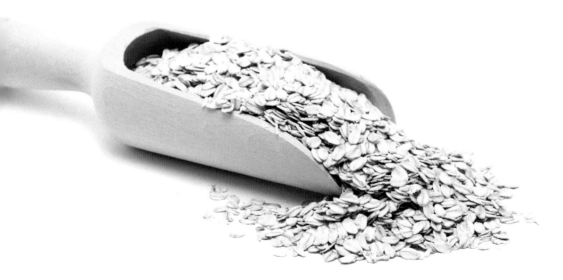

Resources

hese products are available at large natural food stores or online. For further information and recommendations, go to 7DayJust JuiceDiet.com.

CLEANSING PRODUCTS AND SERVICES

Colon Cleansing Products

Bob's Red Mill Organic Whole Ground Flaxseed Meal

NOW Foods Psyllium Husk Powder

RenewLife CleanseMore (capsules include milk of magnesia and can be used as a replacement for it)

RenewLife FiberSmart

Yerba Prima Psyllium Husk Powder

Colon Hydrotherapy

To find a colonic therapist near you, search your local health media or go to: www.i-act.org/IACTSearch.htm

Colonoscopy

www.cdc.gov/cancer/colorectal/basic_info/screening/guidelines.htm

Digestive Enzymes (SEE PAGE 81)

Enzymedica Digest Basic Essential Digestive Enzymes

Nature's Plus Acti-Zyme with Live Food Enzymes FOS & Bioperine

Nature's Sources AbsorbAid Platinum Super Digestive Blend

Herbal Bitters (SEE PAGE 81)

Nature's Answer Bitters with Ginger (alcohol-free)
NatureWorks Swedish Bitters
NOW Foods Digestive Bitters
Planetary Herbals Digestive Grape Bitters
Urban Moonshine Organic Bitters
Wise Woman Herbals Bittersweet Elixir

Mustard Baths

Dr. Singha's Mustard Bath

Probiotics

(AVAILABLE IN NATURAL FOOD STORES)

Bio-K Plus Probiotic Drink (available in rice, soy, or dairy)
NewChapter Probiotic All-Flora
Natural Factors Mega Probiotic Powder
NOW Foods Probiotic Defense
RenewLife Ultimate Flora (30 or 50 billion units per serving)

(AVAILABLE FROM HEALTH PROFESSIONALS OR FROM 7DAYJUSTJUICEDIET.COM)

BioGenesis Pro Flora Intensive (112.5 billion units per serving)
Designs for Health Probiotic Synergy Powder (20 billion units per serving)
Genestra HMF Neuro Powder (12 billion units per serving)
Genestra HMF Super Powder (10 billion units per serving)
Innate Response Formula Flora 50-14 Clinical Strength (50 billion units per serving, 16 strains)
Ther-Biotic Complete Powder (100 billion units per serving, 12 strains)
Sedona Labs Pro IFlora Multi (40 billion units per serving, 16 strains)

Vitamin C (SEE PAGE 68)

NOW Foods Calcium Ascorbate Powder
NOW Foods Magnesium Ascorbate Powder
Solgar Calcium Ascorbate Crystals

Source Naturals Ultimate Ascorbate C Powder

Twinlab Super Ascorbate C

Wheatgrass Juice Products

Sproutman's Wheatgrass Juice Powder and Tablets

Perfect Food RAW Wheat Grass Juice Powder

NOW Foods Wheat Grass Juice Powder

Eclectic Institute Wheat Grass Juice Powder

Vibrant Health USA Field of Greens Powder

Frozen Wheatgrass Juice Extract (through www.Sproutman.com)

DIET

Broth and Bouillon

Vogue Cuisine Instant VegeBase Low-Sodium Soup Base Powder

Marigold Organic Swiss Vegetable Bouillon Cubes

Pacific Foods Organic Vegetable Broth Liquid

Nut and Grain Milks (SUGAR- AND PRESERVATIVE-FREE)

Pacific Foods Organic Almond Milk, Oat Milk, or Hazelnut Milk

Imagine Foods Rice Dream

Vegetable Wash

Beaumont Products Veggie Wash

Fit Fruit and Vegetable Wash

Environne Fruit & Vegetable Wash

SPROUTMAN

Sproutman's 7-Day Just Juice Diet Webinars

7DayJustJuiceDiet.com

Sproutman provides sprouters, organic sprouting seeds, juicers, blenders, dehydrators, kitchen gear, wheatgrass, and courses and books for vibrant health. Visit Sproutman.com

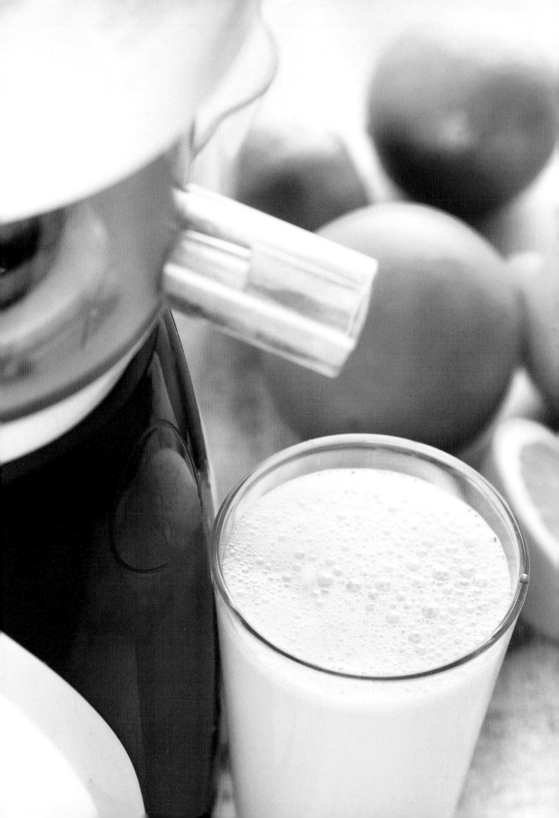

Index

NOTE: Recipe names appear in *italics*. Table references are indicated with a *t*.

A

activated charcoal, 65
acupuncture meridians, 59
aerobic exercise, for detoxification, 54. *see also* exercise
afternoon routine, 48
allergies, 4
Antioxidant Fruit Smoothie, 120
apples
    Cider Vinegar Drink, 61, 112
    Juice, Pineapple-, 106
    juicing with, 35

B

bacteria, good, 24–25, 66
bark chews/gum, 81
Basic Green Smoothie, 118
Basic Plan
    defined, 41, 41*t*
    structure, 40
bathing
    at bedtime, 48–49
    for detoxification, 57–59
    steam baths, 41
bedtime routine, 48–49
beets
    Juice, Sweet, 105
    juicing with, 35
bentonite clay, 64–65
Bentonite-Psyllium Seed Colon Cleanser, 110
bifidobacteria, 25
broths
    Homemade Vegetable, 117

Instant Vegetable, 115
Miso Nori, 116
Simple Miso Soup, 96
brushing, for skin, 56

C

caffeine, eliminating, 12–14
calcium oxalate, 18
Cantaloupe Smoothie, 122
capsules, of probiotics, 50
carrots, juicing, 34–35
Carrot Spinato Juice, 103
catabolic cycle, of exercise, 55
centrifugal juicers, 30
chewing, importance of, 74, 76
chia seeds, 47
citrus juices
    benefits of, 20–21
    citrus juicers, 31, 35
    citrus skins, 32
    Lemon-Ginger Green Juice, 102
    lemon juice, 61
    Lemon Tea, Hot, 113
    vitamin C flush, 68
cleansing drinks. *see also* juicing
    about, 121
    recipes, 111–114
cleanup, of juicers, 35–36
clothing, skin and, 56
coconut, for solid food transition, 78
coffee, eliminating from diet, 12–14
coffee enemas, 64
colon
    colonics, 41, 91

colonoscopy, 67
enemas, 63–64
hydrotherapy, 65–67
colon cleansers
    benefits of, 6, 19, 107
    planning daily routine, 45, 47
    recipes, 107–110
    for solid food transition, 74
    weekly use of, 90
commitment, to cleanse, 9
compresses, hot, 62–63
convenience, of juicers, 31
crucifers, juicing, 17

D

daily routine. *see* planning daily routine
dairy-free diet, 83–84
deep breathing, 82
detoxification, 53–70
    aerobic exercise for, 54
    defined, 3
    exercise for, 5
    extending, beyond juice fast, 83–85, 89–91
    footbaths, 59–60
    for health, 87–91
    hot baths for, 48–49, 57–59
    importance of, 53–54
    for intestines, 64–68
    for liver, 60–64
    lymphatic system and, 55–57
    overall approach to, 54, 57
    special care for mouth, ears, nose, and eyes, 69–70
    for urinary tract, 68–69

diabetes, 10
diary
    planning daily routine, 51, 52t
    recording goals in, 8
digestion
    digestive enzymes for, 81
    restarting, 72–73 (*see also* solid food transition)
    work of, 1
distilled water, 69
Dr. Singha's Mustard Bath, 58–59
doctors, risk evaluation by, 9–10

E
ears, special care for, 69–70
eating, after fasting. *see* solid food transition
effort, juicers and, 32
enemas
    coffee, 64
    colonics *versus*, 66–67
    wheatgrass, 63–64
energy, increasing, 1, 4–5
Energy Lifter Smoothie, 119
enzymes
    production of, 11
    solid food transition and, 80–81
Epsom salt bath, 58–59
evening routine, 48
exercise
    as daily routine, 90
    for detoxification, 5, 62
    muscle strength and, 55
    planning daily routine, 48
    during solid food transition, 82
Expanded Plan, defined, 41, 42t
expectations, for juice fast, 11–14
extraction, with juicers, 30
eyes, special care for, 69–70

F
fasting, benefits of, 1, 3–5. *see also* detoxification; 7-Day Just Juice Diet; solid food transition
fermented foods, 25
fiber
    for detoxification, 64
    planning daily routine, 44
    sources of, 6, 47
financial issues
    juicers, 29–30, 33
    organic foods, 26
flaxseeds
    Colon Cleanser, 108
    for detoxification, 64
    soluble fiber of, 6
fluids. *see also* juicing; water
    daily goal for, 5
    drinks for detoxification, 61–62
flu symptoms, recognizing, 12
foam, in juice, 35
footbaths, for detoxification, 59–60
fruit juices. *see also* recipes
    juicing recommendations, 21
    preparing fruits for, 33–34, 35
    sweet, 20–22
    volume of juice from common fruits and vegetables, 28t

G
garlic, for detoxification, 61
gastrointestinal problems, 3
genetically modified (GMO) foods, 86
ginger
    for detoxification, 61
    Lemon- Green Juice, 102
    Tea, Hot, 114
gluten-free diet, 83
goals, for juice fast, 8–11

grain-free diet, 83
Granny's Green Juice, 104
Grapefruit Liver Cleanser
    daily use of, 89
    as gentle cathartic, 64
    for morning routine, 46
    olive oil in, 19
    recipe, 111
    for solid food transition, 74–75
green juice
    from fresh vegetable juices, 17–18 (*see also* juicing)
    Granny's, 104
    Lemon-Ginger, 102
    from powder, 18, 23–24
    Sproutman's Basic, 97
    Tamari-Garlic, 99

H
"healing crisis," 11–12
health, detoxification for, 87–91. *see also* detoxification; *individual body part names*
herbal bitters, 81
herbal teas, 61, 62
high colonic, 65–57
high-pressure processing (HPP), 89
Homemade Oat Milk, 124
Homemade Vegetable Broth, 117
hot bath
    at bedtime, 48–49
    for detoxification, 57–59
    steam baths, 41
hot beverages. *see also* broths
    about, 22–23
    Ginger Tea, 61, 114
    herbal teas, 61, 62
    Lemon Tea, 113
    tea, 81
hot compresses, 62–63
Hot Ginger Tea, 61, 114
Hot Lemon Tea, 113

hydrotherapy
    colon, 65–67
    hot bath for, 48–49, 57–59

I

Instant Vegetable Broth, 115
insulin dosage, 10
intestines
    detoxification for, 64–68
    size of, 53
inversion exercises, 62
ionic footbath, 60

J

journal. *see* diary
juicers, 29–38
    choosing, 29–33
    storing and transporting
        fresh juice, 36–38
    successful juicing with,
        33–36
juicing, 15–28. *see also* juicers
    colon-cleansing drinks, 19
    components of Just Juice
        Diet, 15, 16
    fruits recommended for, 21
    green juice from powder,
        18, 23–24
    green vegetable juices and
        process of, 17–18
    juice volume from common
        fruits and vegetables,
        28*t*
    optional drinks, 22–23
    organics for, 25–26
    probiotics with, 24–25
    process of, 33–36
    shopping lists, 27
    storing and transporting
        fresh juice, 36–38
    sweet juices and fruit juices,
        20–22
    variety of juices, 20
    vegetables recommended
        for, 18–19
    water, 15–17

K

kale, 17
kidneys
    cleansing of, 7–8
    kidney stones, 18
    urinary tract detoxification,
        68–69
kombucha, 24

L

lactobacillus, 25
laxative. *see* milk of magnesia
leafy vegetables, juicing with,
    34
lemons. *see also* citrus juices
    -Ginger Green Juice, 102
    juicing, 61
    Tea, Hot, 113
Lite Plan, defined, 42, 43*t*
liver
    cleansing benefits, 7
    cleansing drinks for, 19
    detoxification for, 60–64
lungs, detoxification for,
    55–56
lymphatic system, detoxifica-
    tion and, 55–57, 87

M

massage, 62
masticating juicers, 30
meals, resuming. *see* solid
    food transition
menu (sample), for solid food
    transition, 77*t*
metabolism, toxins from, 3
Meyerowitz, Steve
    Water, the Ultimate Cure, 17
    *Wheatgrass: Nature's Finest
        Medicine,* 24
microbiome, 24–25
Mild Spinach Juice, 98
milk of magnesia
    benefits of, 7
    for detoxification, 64
    planning daily routine, 50

Miso Nori Broth, 116
Miso Soup, Simple, 96
morning routine, 46
mouth, special care for, 69–70
mucilage, 6
muscle strength, exercise and,
    55
mustard bath, 58–59

N

nose, special care for, 69–70

O

Oat Milk, Homemade, 124
Oat Milk-Papaya Smoothie, 123
olive oil, 19
organic fruits/vegetables
    benefits of, 25–26
    extended cleansing strategy
        and, 85–86
oxalic acid, 18

P

parsley, 17
perspiration, 56
phytochemicals (plant chemi-
    cals), 1
phytoestrogens (plant estro-
    gens), 3
pineapple, benefits of, 21
Pineapple-Apple Juice, 106
planning daily routine, 39–52
    Basic Plan, defined, 41, 41*t*
    Basic Plan structure, 40
    cleansing schedule, 43–45,
        44*t*
    clearing schedule and, 9
    colon cleansers, 45, 47
    dividing day into five parts,
        45–49
    Expanded Plan, defined,
        41, 42*t*
    Lite Plan, defined, 42, 43*t*
    milk of magnesia, 50
    pre-fast diet, 39–40
    pre-fast recipes, 94–96

probiotics, 50
polyphenols (plant chemicals), 3
pre-fast diet, 39–40
prevention, health and, 88
probiotics
  benefits of, 24–25
  planning daily routine, 50
  for solid food transition, 82
psyllium seeds
  Bentonite- Seed Colon Cleanser, 110
  Colon Cleanser, 109
  for detoxification, 64
  soluble fiber of, 6
pulp, in juice, 36
purgatives, 67

R
raw diet, 83
recipes, 93–124
  about, 93, 108, 121
  Antioxidant Fruit Smoothie, 120
  Apple Cider Vinegar Drink, 112
  Basic Green Smoothie, 118
  Bentonite-Psyllium Seed Colon Cleanser, 110
  Cantaloupe Smoothie, 122
  Carrot Spinato Juice, 103
  Energy Lifter Smoothie, 119
  Flaxseed Colon Cleanser, 108
  Granny's Green Juice, 104
  Grapefruit Liver Cleanser, 111
  Homemade Oat Milk, 124
  Homemade Vegetable Broth, 117
  Hot Ginger Tea, 114
  Hot Lemon Tea, 113
  Instant Vegetable Broth, 115
  Lemon-Ginger Green Juice, 102
  Mild Spinach Juice, 98
  Miso Nori Broth, 116

Oat Milk-Papaya Smoothie, 123
Pineapple-Apple Juice, 106
Psyllium Seed Colon Cleanser, 109
Simple Miso Soup, 96
Simple Salad, 95
Simple Salad Dressing, 94
Spinach-Tomato Juice, 100
Sproutman's Basic Green Juice, 97
Sproutman's V-8 Juice, 101
Sweet Beet Juice, 105
Tamari-Garlic Green Juice, 99
rest, planning for, 51
risk evaluation, 9–10
routing, daily. *see* planning daily routine

S
salads
  Dressing, Simple, 94
  Simple, 95
  solid food transition, 79
sample menu, for solid food transition, 77t
saunas, 41
schedule. *see* planning daily routine
sea vegetables, for pre-fast diet, 39
sediment, straining, 37
self-control, for solid food transition, 78–79
sensitivity, to foods, 4
7-Day Just Juice Diet, 1–14. *see also* detoxification; juicing; planning daily routine; recipes; solid food transition
  benefits of, 1, 3–5
  cleansing with juice, 5–8
  components of, 15, 16
  defined, 2
  expectations for, 11–14
  frequency of, 90, 91

mind-set and goals for, 8–11
smoothies as juice alternative, 14
shopping lists, 27
Simple Miso Soup, 96
Simple Salad, 95
Simple Salad Dressing, 94
skin
  detoxification for, 55–56
  problems affecting, 4
  therapies for cleansing of, 57
smoothies
  Antioxidant Fruit, 120
  Basic Green, 118
  Cantaloupe, 122
  Energy Lifter, 119
  fruits recommended for, 21
  as juice alternative, 14
  Oat Milk-Papaya, 123
  for solid food transition, 76–78
solid food transition, 71–86
  Day 1 (Phase I), 73–76
  Day 2 (Phase II), 76–79, 77t
  Day 3 (Phase III), 79–82
  Day 4 (Phase IV), 82–83
  extending detoxification, 83–85
  organic foods for ongoing detoxification, 85–86
  planning for, 71–73, 73t
  post-fast recipes, 118–124
  pre-fast diet, 39–40
  pre-fast recipes, 94–96
soluble fiber, 6
Soup, Simple Miso, 96. *see also* broths
speed, of juicers, 30–31
spinach
  Carrot Spinato Juice, 103
  Juice, Mild, 98
  juicing, 17
  -Tomato Juice, 100
Sproutman's Basic Green Juice, 97
Sproutman's V-8 Juice, 101
sprouts, 75

steam baths, 41
storage, of fresh juice, 36–38
strength training, 55
sugar, in juices, 20–21, 24
sugar-free diet, 84–85
supplements, abstaining from, 5
support system, 10–11
sweet juices
  about, 20–22
  recipes, 105–106

T
tai chi, 54
Tamari-Garlic Green Juice, 99
tea, 81
temptation, resisting, 76, 81–82
tongue cleaning, 69–70
trampolines, 56, 62
transportation, of fresh juice,
  36–38

U
urinary tract

cleansing of, 7–8
detoxification for, 68–69

V
vegan diet, 83, 84
Vegetable Broth, Instant, 115,
  117
vegetable juices
  green, 17–18
  green, from powder, 23–24
  preparing vegetables for,
    33–35
  recipes, 97–104
  vegetables recommended
    for, 18–19
  volume of juice from com-
    mon fruits and vegeta-
    bles, 28t
vitamin B$_{12}$, 84
vitamin C flush, 68
V-8 Juice, Sproutman's, 101
volume of juice, from common
  fruits and vegetables, 28t

W
water
  avoiding during meals, 80
  benefits of, 15–17
  cleanliness of, 17
  distilled, for urinary tract
    detoxification, 69
  water content of foods, for
    transition to solid foods,
    73
  Water Flush, 16–17, 46
Water, the Ultimate Cure
  (Meyerowitz), 17
weight loss, 3
*Wheatgrass: Nature's Finest
  Medicine* (Meyerowitz),
  24
wheatgrass juice, 23–24,
  63–64

Y
yoga, 54, 62

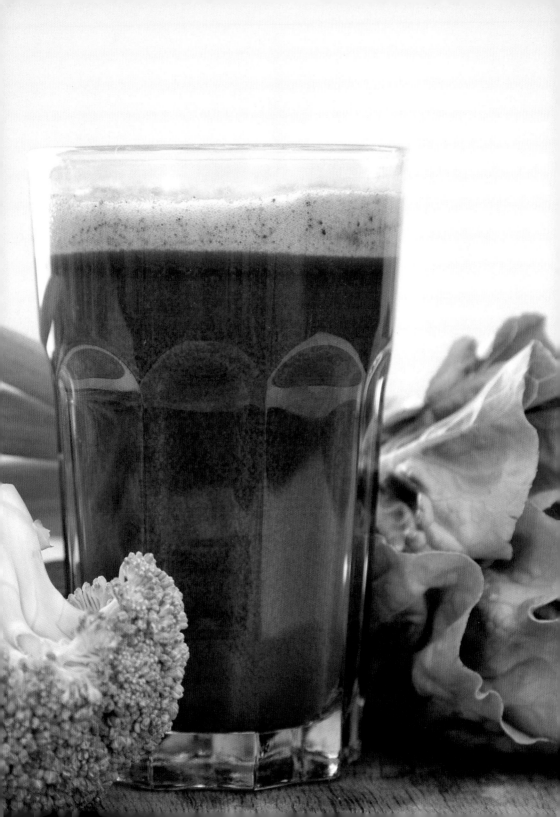

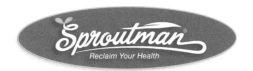

also by Steve Meyerowitz

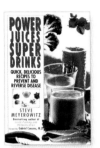

POWER JUICES, SUPER DRINKS

Quick, Delicious Recipes to
Reverse and Prevent Disease

*This is one of the best resource
books on the power of foods and
herbs that I own.*
—Ayesha Rognlie, ND

$16.00 ● ISBN 978-1-57566-528-3

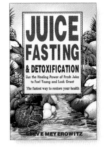

JUICE FASTING & DETOXIFICATION

Use the Healing Power
of Fresh Juice to Feel Young
and Look Great

Includes illustrations, photos,
and charts.

$10.95 ● ISBN 978-1-87873-665-9

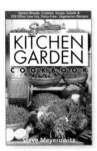

SPROUTMAN'S KITCHEN GARDEN COOKBOOK

Create breads, cookies, soups,
salads, and 250 other low-fat,
dairy-free vegetarian recipes
with sprouts.

$14.95 ● ISBN 978-1-87873-686-4

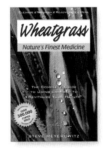

WHEATGRASS: NATURE'S FINEST MEDICINE

Get the complete guide to using
various forms of grasses and grass
juices to improve your health.

$14.95 ● ISBN 978-1-87873-698-7

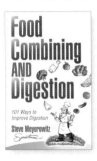

FOOD COMBINING and DIGESTION

101 Ways to Improve Digestion

Eat better to feel better.
Includes illustrations and charts.

$9.95 ● ISBN 978-1-87873-677-2

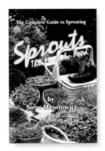

SPROUTS: THE MIRACLE FOOD

The Complete Guide to Sprouting

Sprouts are the world's most
nutritious vegetables.

Includes charts, seed resources,
illustrations, and photos.

$12.95 ● ISBN 978-1-87873-604-8

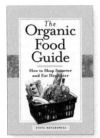

THE ORGANIC FOOD GUIDE

Organic foods boost nutrition,
flavor, and health at every age.
Learn about pesticides, labels
and claims, and shopping wisely.
Illustrated with photos and
charts.

$8.95 ● ISBN 978-0-7627-3069-8

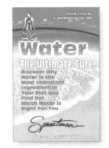

WATER: THE ULTIMATE CURE

Discover why water is the most
important ingredient in your diet
and find out which water is right
for you.

You are not sick, you are thirsty!
—F. Batmanghelidj, MD.

$7.95 ● ISBN 978-1-87873-620-8

GO TO ***Sproutman.com***

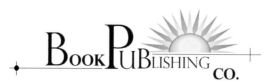

BookPublishing Co.

books that educate, inspire, and empower

To find your favorite vegetarian and soyfood products online, visit:
healthy-eating.com

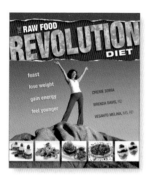

**The Raw Food
Revolution Diet**
*Cherie Soria,
Brenda Davis, RD,
Vesanto Melina, MS, RD*
978-1-57067-185-2 • $21.95

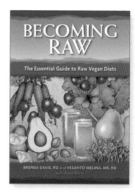

Becoming Raw
*Brenda Davis, RD,
Vesanto Melina, MS, RD,
with Rynn Berry*
978-1-57067-238-5 • $24.95

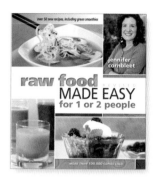

**Raw Food Made Easy
for 1 or 2 People**
REVISED EDITION
Jennifer Cornbleet
978-1-57067-273-6 • $19.95

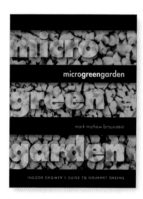

Microgreen Garden
Mark M. Braunstein
978-1-57067-294-1 • $14.95

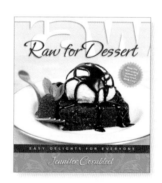

Raw for Dessert
Jennifer Cornbleet
978-1-57067-236-1 • $14.95

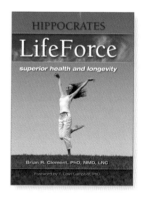

Hippocrates LifeForce
*Brian Clement,
PhD, NMD, LNC*
978-1-57067-249-1 • $14.95

Purchase these health titles and cookbooks from your local bookstore or natural food store,
or you can buy them directly from:

Book Publishing Company • P.O. Box 99 • Summertown, TN 38483 • 800-695-2241
Please include $3.95 per book for shipping and handling.